Coconut Oil
Miracle or Myth?

JEAN ARMSTRONG

Hula Books
Delhi ~ Canada

Published by Hula Books (Canada)
Suite #872, 693 Peel Street
Delhi N4B2H3

Canada – USA – UK – India – Ireland
New Zealand - Australia – South Africa

www.hulaboks.com

Printed in The United States of America

Book Design by Laura Childs of HulaBooks
Edited by Veronica Childs

ISBN-10: 1497331536
ISBN-13: 978-1497331532

DEDICATION

Written with appreciation for
every child, teen, and adult
who questions everything
and seeks alternatives
to society's norm.

TABLE OF CONTENTS

ACKNOWLEDGMENTS

To the scientists, doctors, biologists, chemists, lab teams, funding corporations, and private companies that investigate, share, and continue the research on coconut oil.

Papers and articles used for research date back to 1960. While newer research and studies are prominent within, acknowledgments are given to the pioneers in the industry and the most prolific publishers of theory.

Please contact the publisher if you feel any name or any legitimate research should be added to this book.

Prof. Dr. Jon J. Kabara (United States of America) – performed the original seminal research regarding certain fatty acids (FAs) and how their derivatives can have adverse effects on various micro-organisms.

J. C. Hierholzer (United States of America)
– Virology Scientist

Mary Gertrude Enig, PhD (United States of America)
- Nutritionist

Bruce Fife (United States of America)
– Author of over 20 books

Dr. Conrado S. Dayrit (Philippines)
– Doctor and Scientist, Professor of Pharmacology

INTRODUCTION

"Mom, it itches!" "Rub some coconut oil on it."

"I'm breaking out." "Put some coconut oil on it."

"I need to lose weight..." "Take a tablespoon of coconut oil..."

For the last 20 years, coconut oil has been our first line of defense against illness, a cure for many irritations, and one of the first ingredients we reach for when cooking. The oil is held in such high regard in our home that our children and their friends now call me The Coconut Mama.

Mainstream media would have you believe that this humble oil is a super food; a healer of miraculous magnitude. This book has been written to set the record straight.

The surface truth is that the oil is as versatile as it is valuable.

It will exceed your expectations as a restorative; from your head to your toes, inside and out. It can also be beneficial to pets and some livestock. In the kitchen coconut oil can replace butter in nearly every recipe and excels as a cooking oil for sautes and fried foods.

As for coconut oil's medicinal properties, it can help you lose weight, increase energy, strengthen your immune system, regulate blood sugar, fight acne, and repair a sluggish metabolism. Research studies and personal testimonies on using coconut oil to prevent cancer, to treat HIV, and to slow the progression of

Alzheimer's - plus multiple other diseases - abound. We will look at many of these claims in later chapters.

Together we will investigate the basis for the miracle claims, and we will debunk the myths. While some are proven, many are still being researched.

Since you've chosen this book above all others on coconut oil, I'll assume you're looking for answers. You've read or heard about the miracle cures of coconut oil. You want to know if they are founded in research or it is nothing but media hype. Uncovering the answers for you - for all of us - has been my quest in writing this book.

Stick with me. By the time you've finished this chapter you'll understand that the real secret to these claims lay in the uncommon composition of the oil.

You'll find ample citations and links to legitimate research supporting the claims.

You'll know why you are only just hearing about the powers of coconut oil today – even though many cultures have been using it for thousands of years. You'll also see the devastating loss of health in those cultures once they switched over to our Western diet.

First though, let's explore the wonderful properties of this oil.

[1]

COCONUT OIL: A MIRACLE CURE?

Coconut oil does has incredible restorative and healing properties, but is it a miracle cure? A modern medical discovery for all things that ail us? Or is the hype (seen on television news, talk shows and web sites) little more than the marketing babble of snake oil salesmen?

Here's the skinny. The proven preventative and restorative powers of coconut oil are that it is:

- an anti-viral
- an anti-bacterial
- an anti-fungal
- an anti-protozoan
- an anti-microbial
- rich in anti-oxidants (therefore anti-carcinogenic)
- food that can be used by the brain, and
- is supportive to bodily systems and functions

At first blush it seems preposterous that one simple oil could have so many virtues.

Many answers to the oil's virtuosity can be found in history. Naturopaths, Ayurvedic, and alternative medicine practitioners have been using coconut oil for eons. For these practitioners, tales of cures and disease remission are commonplace.

It is reasonable to look to ancient practices when our specialists can't cure our disease. Modern medicine is founded in ancient cures, after all.

While many medical professionals, clinics, and scientists are taking a closer look at coconut oil's power to cure, more of each are needed. The growing list of testimonials and news stories - from those who have been healed or are in remission - is helping in this regard.

In North America, we need to see scientific proof and the underlying research before we'll be swayed by claims of miraculous healing. This is true until we are desperate; the time at which modern medicine has failed to cure us.

We may take pride and believe in Western medical practices, but it is important to note that on a global scale we are neither leaders in health, nor wellness, nor longevity.

Alternative medicine has much to teach us.

Within these pages you will find references and treatments that require a leap of faith. This is particularly true of claims that are without extensive supporting research. While I considered leaving those remedies on the editing floor, to do so would be a disservice.

My goal is to empower you. To inspire you to become a champion of your own health. I will attempt to do so in the most honest, upright fashion possible.

Ayurvedic Medicine

Ayurvedic medicine is native to India and documented from as early as 100BC. To Westerners, Ayurvedic medicine is classified as ancient or alternative. Treatments and lifestyle is still taught, respected, and practiced today.

According to Ayurvedic teachings, oils support natural immunity, fight illness, and protect good health. Various oils are prescribed in a pure state as well as used as a carrier base for herbal remedies.

I'll teach you (in layman's terms) about the composition of coconut oil and how our body uses and reacts to it. This knowledge acquisition is the truest path to believing or debunking any 'miraculous claim' that comes your way.

I will not be filling up pages with botany and biology. This book is intended to be a working manual for the layperson, not a scientific journal.

As we examine each claim in following chapters I will do my best to explain why or how coconut oil might help you or your family. Wherever possible I will reference and/or link to legitimate research studies. Should you choose to delve deeper into the science behind a claim, you will have it at your fingertips.

I assume that you are in good health and are on a mission to maintain that state. Therefore you will find uses for coconut oil - from replacing the chemical-laden personal care products in your cupboard, to information on healing, supporting, or alleviating the symptoms of, illness and disease.

Finally, since coconut oil is a food, I'll share some of my favorite coconut oil recipes with you.

To date, science has proven that coconut oil:

- supports thyroid and adrenal glands, which affect hormones and metabolism;
- bypasses the pancreas, which improves insulin resistance;
- provides quick energy, which makes it an invaluable appetite suppressant;
- provides food for the brain, which increases clarity and focus;
- creates a healthier HDL to LDL (cholesterol) ratio, which supports heart and arteries;
- improves the absorption of fat-soluble vitamins and nutrients;[1]
- protects against viral and bacterial infections and disease;
- manages over-population of microbial, parasitic, protozoic, and fungi growth;
- protects against oxidation at the cellular level;
- moisturizes, rejuvenates, and protects skin, hair, and nails; and
- attacks the cellular membrane of life-threatening virus and bacteria.

These are high claims indeed for an oil pressed out of a nut!

Each has been proven on some level. Research is on-going. Research is also on-going on the theory that all saturated fats cause heart disease; a 'truth' we have bought into for over half a century.

---

1 Vitamins A, D, E, K; all B vitamins; beta-carotene, CoQ10, calcium and magnesium, lycopene, as well as some amino acids.

Rants, Stance, and Reasoning

While coconut oil seems to be the newest miracle cure for whatever ails you, Westerners were once large consumers of the oil. Just ask your grandmother. Coconut oil may have been a common staple in her cupboard too, an easy substitution for butter, lard or shortening.

As a child I explored cooking alone. Our kitchen was well stocked by a career-focused mother.

> **"As for butter versus margarine, I trust the cows more than chemists."**
> Joan Dye Gussow

Since it was the early 70s, there wasn't much that I'd eat from the cupboards. Packaged items and dinners tasted of chemicals. Even FDA-approved additives in canned soup turned my stomach. Chemical tastes would linger on my tongue for hours after eating those 'foods'.

Coconut oil was on our shelf. It was an oddity. The label read "oil", but it looked like lard. It would melt instantly on the tongue, but lacked flavor.[2]

As the years passed my taste buds adapted. I grew to eat what friends and family ate, lost my sensitivity to unnatural flavors and chemicals, and gained weight as a result.

The acceptance of those additives increased my waistline, slowed my metabolism, and muddied my concentration.

---

2 In retrospect I believe this was an RBD (refined, bleached and deodorized) coconut oil.

In the last 15 years I've managed to turn that back around. With the initial help of coconut oil as a detox agent, plus returning to more natural foods, good health has returned.

Unnatural processing and additives should not have a place in our sustenance. There are ample chemical toxins – sprayed on our vegetables, fed to our livestock, pumped into the air we breathe, added to our water supply – causing enough damage to our bodies. Can we afford to add insult to injury by consuming convenience foods?

We all believe that a busy life demands convenience foods; that they are a necessary evil - but at what cost? Fillers, chemical additives and compounds, or messing with whole foods at a molecular level, is at the root of many ills.

Coming to light are the sober implications of eating factory-made foodstuff. Obesity, death and life-threatening illness' are on the rise.

More Than Our Food Is Killing Us

Until now we haven't had to worry about products being safe. Our government analyzes and approves all new items introduced to the marketplace, publishes guidelines for a healthy diet, and monitors prescription medications carefully.

Do you agree?

The sad truth is that we have been lulled into a false sense of security. Until the age of the internet, few of us knew we had options. Few knew that we could and should question the science behind every item formulated as food, medicine, or personal care.

Our skin is our body's largest organ. Everything we put onto it leeches into our bloodstream and subsequently, our cells. Lotions and shampoos are no different from food in this regard. If it isn't safe to eat, we shouldn't be dousing our bodies with it.

It took the birth of my first child for me to fully understand that concept. In my arms, a pink bundle of tender skin that I had sworn to protect. On the shelves around me were specialty skin creams and shampoos, medicated creams, no-tear formulas and ointments -- all of unknown ingredients.

I couldn't do it. I could not affect such a pure and healthy life with products from a chemistry lab.

Research for healthier alternatives began at the health food store. Store staff introduced me to natural care products while educating me on the versatility and safety of coconut oil.

Knowledge plus simplicity affords peace of mind.

Switching out products made logical sense. Coconut oil was already a main ingredient in skin care products, we were just leaving behind the chemicals and fragrance. Simply getting back to basics.

This was also a frugal choice. Even if coconut oil tripled in price, we'd still be saving money.

Coconut oil is also proactive to good health; a prime concern when raising children. Why wait for illness or infection (caused by germs, bacteria and virus) when you can support an immune system that will block harmful organisms?

A Coconut Oil Challenge for You

While it did take a few years for "put some coconut oil on it" to become a theme phrase in our house, our use has since expanded. Outside of food, medicinal and personal care, we also use the oil on pets and some livestock.

I'd like to challenge you to start using coconut oil in at least 5 ways by the time you finish reading this book. You'll find many reasonable purposes and examples following in later chapters. My hunch is that you'll be like many of the people I've convinced in the past – once you start using it, you'll never be without it on your shelf.

If you'd like to share your favorite way or how you used coconut oil for healing, your story could be added to a future edition of this book. Send us an email at editor@hulabooks.com.

[3]

COMPOSITION OF COCONUT OIL

Coconut oil is classified as a vegetable oil. It has the highest count of saturated fatty acids of any other oil.

The major difference between coconut oil and other saturated fats is where we discover the benefits.

Sixty-two percent of coconut oil's fat consists of medium-chain fatty acids.[3]

Medium-chain fatty acids make the oil easier for our bodies to convert to energy. We do so nearly as fast as we convert simple carbohydrates, but without the harmful spikes in blood sugar.

Composition of Coconut Oil	(% by weight)	
Saturated fatty acids		91
Mono-unsaturated fatty acids		5
Polyunsaturated fatty acids (total)		3
Omega-3 Linolenic acid		-
Omega 6 Linoleic acid	2	
Oleic acid		6

---

3 Remaining composition is: short-chain fatty acids, 0.5%; long-chain fatty acids, 37.5%.

For decades we have been told that all saturated fats are unhealthy.

If this is true how is it that coconut oil has helped so many North Americans lose weight, repair their metabolism, and improve overall health?

How is it that some cultures – traditionally eating large amounts of coconut oil (Sri Lanka, Thailand, the Philippines, and the Pacific islands) – have a relatively low incidence of heart disease?[4]

Low, that is, until we influenced their culture with our Western dietary standards. Once the swap from coconut oil to other oils were made, their statistics rose to match ours.

Coconut oil was once a common ingredient in packaged foods. Products containing it had a long shelf life and the fat maintained a stable consistency. When we decided that saturated fat was unhealthy, hydrogenated vegetable oils replaced coconut oil. Hydrogenated oils also maintained their consistency on the shelf, but that is their only virtue.

Hydrogenated oils have been linked to Alzheimer's, ADHD, high cholesterol, atherosclerosis and more. Compare that, with proof in later chapters, to coconut oil's restorative qualities.

Dig deeper into the differences between oils and you'll discover some heady controversy and conspiracy theories.

We shall get to all of it.

---

4 "Study Shows Heart Disease Absent in Coconut Eating Population", Department of Agriculture, Philippine Coconut Authority, http://www.pca.da.gov.ph/heartdisease.php

Coconut Oil's Fatty Acids

This saturated fat is a good dietary fat. What scientists know today about the human body, paired with the underlying science of this fat's composition, make adding coconut oil to your diet as smart as choosing olive oil over corn oil.

Setting all that aside, let's look at the fatty acid composition of coconut oil. These acids present as uncommon, medium-chain triglycerides (MCTs).

What's A Triglyceride?

A triglyceride is made up of 3 fatty acids connected to a glyceride molecule. As our body breaks these down they become diglycerides (two fatty acid connected to the glyceride), monoglycerides (one fatty acid connected to the glyceride), and free fatty acids.

MCTs are easily converted into energy. They are largely responsible for the weight loss and metabolism-related claims of coconut oil.

There's more to love about MCTs though.

Coconut oil's MCTs contain multiple acids (up to 10 known types) which include lauric acid, caprylic acid, capric acid, caproic acid, palmitic acid, and myristic acid.

While all have value, the most prevalent and researched are lauric (approximately 44%), myristic (approximately 16.8%) and capric/caprylic (approximately 6-7%).[5]

_____

5   Composition percentages will vary.

Lauric acid is a miracle in its own right. It is found only in a few natural oils and milks. Of milks, human breast milk has the highest concentration (approximately 6.2%), followed by goat's milk (approximately 3.1%) and lastly, cow's milk (approximately 2.9%).[6]

The fact that human breast milk is naturally high in lauric acid sparked a few 'light bulb moments' in this mom's brain. Nutritious, easily digestible, and beneficial to life outside the womb. A life that is rife with bacteria, fungi, viruses and parasites. Just like a mom, lauric acid is poised to protect us from all four perils!

On its own, lauric acid is used in oral and topical medications. It is prescribed in various forms for influenza, swine and avian flu, common colds and cold sores, genital herpes (HSV), genital warts (HPV) and even to manage the viral load of HIV/AIDS sufferers.

Lauric acid based medicines also treat bronchitis, gonorrhea, ringworm, yeast infections and chlamydia. It fights the infection caused by the protozoan parasite Giardia lamblia – one of the most insidious infections of our time.

Lauric acid has been the star of the show in hundreds of important research studies.

Does it help with acne?[7]

Will it cure respiratory disease?[8]

Can it prevent cavities?[9]

---

6   Composition percentages will vary.

7   "Antimicrobial property of lauric acid against Propionibacterium acnes: its therapeutic potential for inflammatory acne vulgaris" (2009) http://www.ncbi.nlm.nih.gov/pubmed/19387482

8   "In Vitro and In Vivo Evaluations of the Activities of Lauric Acid Monoester Formulations against Staphylococcus aureus", (2005), http://aac.asm.org/content/49/8/3187

9   "Effect of Oil-Pulling on Oral Microorganisms in Biofilm Models" (2010-2011), http://asiaph.org/admin/img_topic/6096Sroisiri.pdf

Will it kill helicobacter pylori?[10]

The list of studies touch upon nearly every illness that affects modern man.

Why are scientists so interested in lauric acid and what makes it so effective?

Introducing Monolaurin

As discussed in the sidebar above, when we consume a triglyceride our body breaks it down into free fatty acids, diglycerides, and monoglycerides. The monoglyceride of lauric acid is monolaurin.[11]

Monolaurin has been used for decades as a surfactant in cosmetics and in deodorant.

What you may appreciate most about monolaurin is that it has anti-microbial[12] properties.

The term anti-microbial covers a wide spectrum of micro-organism inhibitors including anti-bacterial, anti-fungal, anti-viral, and anti-parasitic.

It gets better.

Monolaurin also stimulates the production of white blood cells, specifically T cells. T cells attack anything that is foreign to the body which includes cancerous cells.

10 "Susceptibility of Helicobacter pylori to Bactericidal Properties of Medium-Chain Monoglycerides and Free Fatty Acid", (1995), http://aac.asm.org/content/40/2/302.full.pdf

11 Monolaurin can also be purchased as a stand-alone supplement and is used in many commercial products.

12 Penicillin was created from the discovery of a naturally occurring anti-microbial. http://en.wikipedia.org/wiki/Antimicrobial

Therefore, as well as fighting, curing, or protecting us against infection, monolaurin also supports the production of our own defence mechanisms.

How Monolaurin Attacks Virus and Bacteria

This little monoglyceride is one tough cookie.

Monolaurin busts through the cellular membrane of some lipid-encased pathogens (fat-enveloped "germs" that cause disease in the human body). The exposed pathogen can neither replicate nor thrive.

More recent evidence suggests that monolaurin interferes with the signal transduction required in pathogenic cell replication. In either case, if a pathogen cannot replicate then it cannot overtake your body and make you sick.

A research paper published in the Journal of Food Safety showed that monolaurin was effective at killing 14 RNA and DNA lipid-encased viruses - shown on the next page.[13]

Even the healthiest among us would suffer if infected with some of these viruses, but for those already suffering with a compromised immune system the effects can be deadly. The same can be said of the lipid-coated bacteria coconut oil has proven to be effective against.

Of special interest regarding monolaurin are the hundreds of unsolicited personal reviews and testimonies. Where most drugs are overwhelmed with chronic complaints and poor ratings, reviews on drugs containing monolaurin are largely favorable.

---

13 "In Vitro Effects of Monolaurin Compounds on Enveloped RNA and DNA Viruses", 1982, http://onlinelibrary.wiley.com/doi/10.1111/j.1745-4565.1982.tb00429.x/abstract

Lipid-Coated Viruses (LCV)

- HIV-1 / HIV+
- Measles
- HSV-1 / HSV-2 / Herpes Viridae
- Human Lymphotropic Viruses (type 1)
- Vesicular Stomatitis Virus (VSV)
- Visna Virus
- Cytomegalovirus
- Epstein-Barr Virus
- Influenza
- Leukemia
- Pneumonovirus
- Sarcoma
- Syncytial
- Rubeola

Lipid-Coated Bacteria (LCB)

- Listeria monocytogenes
- Helicobacter pylori
- Hemophilus influenzae
- Staphylococcus aureus
- Streptococcus agalactiae
- Groups A, B, F & G streptococci

Monolaurin isn't just medicine, it is preventative medicine. It doesn't just kill harmful microbes, it prevents attacks and corrects imbalances. And while it may not cure every ill, it can certainly make us healthier by decreasing our viral load.

Those fighting off disease caused from bacteria and viruses have asked: "Can I treat myself? What is the standard treatment protocol?"

It is my stance that without proper training, few of us can treat ourselves. All aspects of an illness must be considered in conjunction with medical history, age, weight, and current environment.

A medical practitioner, specialist or naturopathic doctor is the best person to turn to for advice on these matters – not something you'd read in a book or on a blog.

To provide an idea of what treatment looks like, Dr. Sherry Rogers suggests that "two capsules of monolaurin (300 mgs) are often taken three times a day at the first sign of infection and continued...until the virus is completely gone."[14]

While sharing such advice without a pre-consultation may seem reckless on Dr. Rogers' part – especially in regards to life-threatening illness – it does provide a starting point for a naturopathic physician's research, or as your opening line with a professional.

Remember though that it is the reduction of viral load that is on the table for discussion, not a cure.[15]

Dr. Rogers' suggestion is to take the supplements until "the virus is completely gone" which may not be possible for all patients, especially those with compromised immunity.

To address the next question that is sure to come: "How much coconut oil will I need to ingest to receive that much monolaurin?", there is no easy answer. Remember that monolaurin is the monoglyceride of lauric acid. Too many natural variables make an exact recommendation unlikely.[16]

---

14 "The High Blood Pressure Hoax", (1st edition, 2005), Sherry A. Rogers, M.D.

15 Personal testimonies can be found through a good Google search.

16 On average, 50 ml (3.4 tbsp) of coconut oil contains 20-25 grams lauric acid – what this converts to as monolaurin however is undocumented.

Should you choose to take them, monolaurin capsules are inexpensive. Ninety 300mgs capsules sell for less than $20 USD online.

Lauric Acid and Cholesterol

While the saturated fat and heart disease debate is still fresh in your mind, it is important to clear up the correlation between coconut oil and cholesterol.

Lauric acid does increase total serum cholesterol, but the main increase is to HDL (high-density lipoprotein) which is the good blood cholesterol.[17]

Early studies also suggest that coconut oil, (when added regularly to a balanced diet), might also lower serum cholesterol by converting ingested cholesterol to pregnenolone[18] instead of packing it away as cholesterol.

How or why would this happen? Through lauric acid's support of thyroid functions.

When the thyroid is at optimum health, the production of pregnenolone and progesterone increase. These two hormones protect our bodies. Their job is to function as an antioxidant, anti-seizure, anti-toxin, anti-clot, and anti-carcinogenic.[19] Inadvertently they are also responsible for brain and bone health.

---

17 "Effects of dietary fatty acids and carbohydrates on the ratio of serum total to HDL cholesterol and on serum lipids and apolipoproteins: a meta-analysis of 60 controlled trials", American Journal of Clinical Nutrition, 2003, http://ajcn.nutrition.org/content/77/5/1146

18 A steroid hormone, with ketone groups, synthesized in the brain. Currently being tested for memory function.

19 Ray Peat, Ph.D. in Biology with specialization in physiology, 2003, http://raypeat.com/articles/articles/coconut-oil.shtml

While I'm over-simplifying the effect of lauric acid on cholesterol, the end result is still clear. With approximately half of coconut oil's fatty acid being represented as lauric acid – replacing some dietary fat with a saturated fat like coconut oil could actually lower your risk of heart disease, not increase it.

Medium-Chain Triglycerides

Finally, we need to look at how our body converts coconut oil's fatty acids into energy.

To recap: Most saturated fats are made of large-chain fatty acids. Coconut oil is made of about 65% medium-chain fatty acids. These acids are contained within medium-chain triglycerides (MCTs) which our bodies further break down into diglycerides, monoglycerides, and free fatty acids.

MCTs are quickly absorbed by the liver where some will be converted into ketone bodies. This process completely bypasses the pancreas and digestive system and ketones are immediately released into the bloodstream to be used as energy.[20]

You can truly appreciate the beauty of MCTs when you compare the above conversion to our standard food-to-energy conversion – turning food first to glucose before the body can utilize the energy. That longer route also determines how the energy will be used. In most of us – sedentary and already heavier than is healthy – that glucose will be stored in our tissues and organs as fat.

The conversion of MCTs to ketones hold the keys to correcting or resetting metabolism, supporting brain function and keeping other organs healthy. Ketones are often put to task as fuel for the

---

20 The liver is also capable of converting other fats to ketones, but will do so only when carbohydrates are kept extremely low in the diet (quite uncommon for most of us in North America).

brain when glucose levels are low, or the brain is incapable of converting glucose (due to disease or dysfunction).

Scientists and medical teams have studied the effects of a ketone based (ketogenic) diet for the last 80+ years. The diet was originally created as a way to reduce the frequency of epileptic seizures in children, it is now being considered as a way to slow degenerative brain disease.

The ketogenic diet is high-fat, low-carbohydrate, with only adequate amounts of protein. The diet forces the body into a state of ketosis, burning existing and ingested fats rather than glucose – all while supporting brain function.

Where once all we had was promise, ongoing research has begun to provide some proof. New research on the affects of MCTs and Alzheimer's, dementia, cancer, lymphoma, fibromyalgia, diabetes, chronic fatigue, lupus, jaundice, cystic fibrosis, and pancreatic insufficiency are all in the works.

[4]

FAT AND OILS PRIMER

Dietary fats provide nutrients that our bodies convert to energy. All fats aid in the absorption of fat-soluble vitamins.

Fats are generally classified as saturated or unsaturated but as you'll see in the list on the following pages, fats have a percentage of both types.

Saturated Fat

At room temperature, saturated fat is a solid. It is found mostly in animal-based foods (dairy products, poultry, fish, pork, beef, etc.) and tropical nut oils (coconut and palm).

Saturated fatty acids are comprised of three subgroups; short-, medium-, and long-chain fatty acids. Each subgroup has different metabolic, biological and pharmacological functions. Medium chain fatty acids are found exclusively in lauric oils (palm and coconut).

Government-issued nutrition guidelines recommend that no more than 10% of daily calories should come from saturated fat.

Unsaturated Fat

At room temperature, unsaturated fat is liquid. It is found in plant-based foods (soybean, corn, sunflower, etc.).

Monounsaturated fat and polyunsaturated fats are sub-types of unsaturated fat. Omega-3 and Omega-6 fatty acids are found in polyunsaturated fats. Omega-9 is found in monounsaturated fats.

Trans-Fat

Trans-fats are a man-made creation. Using them to the extent that we have is the result of early research stating that saturated fats were unhealthy.

These fats are created by hydrogenating unsaturated fats – manipulating molecules of a liquid oil so that it acts more like a solid or semi-solid fat. The inclusion of these fats in a packaged product gave it a longer, more stable shelf life; but put a shorter expiry date on the humans who consume them. (Remember that these hydrogenated oils have been linked to Alzheimer's, ADHD, high cholesterol and more.)

At some point each of us needs to look at our diet to assess the quantity, quality, and types of fat that are best for us. A doctor or naturopathic practitioner may guide you toward a healthful diet but I urge you to continue in your research of fats and oils. I've supplied a few good books on this topic in the final chapter.

Personally, I won't eat a hydrogenated (trans) fat of any quantity if I can avoid it. This is more of a challenge than it appears. Take a look at the labels of food in your cupboards. Even simple condiments (mayonaisse, salad dressings, etc.) are made with vegetable oils that have been processed, hydrogenated and altered from their natural state.

Regarding saturated fat intake, I'd estimate my diet to be about 12-14% during winter months, 7-10% in the summer.

I can be an extremist about the smoke point of all fats and oils when cooking.

In my cupboard you'll only find virgin olive and coconut oils. In the fridge; butter and lard. We don't buy lard, we collect it from the bacon we cure at home.

For reference, here are our most commonly used fats, showing the percentage of saturated to unsaturated content per 100 grams.

Butter

Saturated fat	63 g
Polyunsaturated fat	26 g
Mononunsaturated fat	4 g

Coconut Oil

Saturated fat	86 g
Polyunsaturated fat	1.8 g
Monounsaturated fat	6 g

Corn Oil

Saturated fat	13 g
Polyunsaturated fat	55 g
Monounsaturated fat	28 g

Lard

Saturated fat	39 g
Polyunsaturated fat	45 g
Mononunsaturated fat	11 g

Olive Oil

Saturated fat	14 g
Polyunsaturated fat	11 g
Monounsaturated fat	73 g

Palm Oil

Saturated fat	49 g
Polyunsaturated fat	9 g
Monounsaturated fat	37 g

Sunflower Seed Oil

Saturated fat	13 g
Polyunsaturated fat	36 g
Monounsaturated fat	46 g

Soybean Oil (hydrogenated)

Saturated fat	21 g
Polyunsaturated fat	0.4g
Mononunsaturated fat	73g

Soybean Oil (unhydrogenated)

Saturated fat	16 g
Polyunsaturated fat	58 g
Mononunsaturated fat	23 g

[5]

YOUR COUNTRY OR YOUR HEALTH

In earlier chapters we touched upon a few healthy body functions that – should they become imbalanced – may cause cancer, brain degeneration, and organ damage. We also looked at a few ways regularly including coconut oil in the diet might help reverse or repair past damage.

If damage has already begun due to diet, most of us know it was our preconceived notions on fats and oils that are to blame. Saturated fats, we have been told, will clog our arteries. Saturated fats will kill us.

Those notions came from the media and from our doctors. Doctors were following government's published nutrition standards. Governments – who have spent large fortunes of tax-payers money on research to ensure their countrymen remain healthy.

Since we have followed those standards and now suffer the consequences, we can't help but wonder if there was an alternate agenda.

Without trying to sway you in any particular direction, what follows is the most believed conspiracy theory, plus facts from published scientific literature. Whenever possible I've provided links to the full published study.

I am neither a doctor nor a scientist but I have spent countless hours pouring over research studies. The testing methods of those studies vary using in vivo (humans), in vivo (animals), and in vitro (test tube). Nearly all blow government published nutrition guidelines regarding fats to smithereens.

Fats, Oils & Big Business

Perhaps you are wondering how North American culture got to where we are today regarding oils, national nutritional guidelines, obesity, and modern day disease?

A lot of us do.

I'm not keen on spreading conspiracy theories or ranting about politicians in bed with corporate sponsors. This chapter therefore, may spark more questions than provide answers.

I agree, the next page's concept is trite, abstract, highly conspiratorial, and judgmental. Yet when you look at how a government agency took the inconclusive results of a good scientist's experiments on fats; how that agency might have recognized the national economic impact; the conspiracy grows easier to believe.

Even more controversial is that the same agency pumping and promoting the "all saturated fats are bad" campaign, also ignored all subsequent experiments on how our bodies use fat.

Why we ever decided to trust a government agency with our health is beyond me!

Does a government office care about the health and longevity of taxpayers?

Not likely.

The longer a taxpayer lives the harder they are on the national debt. Senior citizens collect on pensions, money that government offices spent long ago.

Governments manage natural resources and money.

Edible oils are big business. From 1910-1970 the consumption of processed and refined vegetable oils rose by 60%.

An Abstract Concept

Every mother that has ever struggled financially knows that she can feed her children by either (a) finding suitable food to grow on her land, or (b) buying the cheapest food available.

Countries know this as well.

Decades ago, in a government office somewhere, there was a decision to be made.

"We need more taxpayers. How will we feed a growing population in a way that keeps people working and wealth within our borders?"

What grows easily and well here?

What is cheap to produce?

"We will sell them on that, then!"

And the national nutrition guidelines were born.

The global vegetable oil market is now poised to reach $91.4 billion by 2017.[21]

There is much at stake. Making choices about dietary fats affects both personal health and the global economy.

Who Stands To Gain?

"North America alone, human consumption of fats and oils adds up to 10 million tonnes each year."[22]

It is a widespread belief that national nutrition guidelines weren't based on studies promoting health, but publicity campaigns promoting soybeans and rapeseed (used for canola oil) – the vegetables used for oil that grow easily on our soil.

Soybean and canola oil have been in the top 3 most popular oils worldwide since 2004 – perhaps longer. The United States is the largest producer of soybean oil. Canada is the largest producer of canola oil. Two western countries – the originators of expensive nutrition research (or publicity campaigns depending on how you want to look at it). Also the originators of the western diet that is killing us off.

The truth can be seen in national health results on both sides of North America's border.

Statistics seldom lie.

Heart disease and other degenerative diseases have increased. Diabetes is on the rise. Obesity is now an epidemic across North

21 "Global Vegetable Oil Market (Edible & Industrial), by Types, Application, Geography & Extraction Methods-Forecasts up to 2017" http://www.marketsandmarkets.com/Market-Reports/vegetable-oil-394.html

22 "The Business of Fats and Oils, Fats That Heal, Fats That Kill", pp 90, (1993) Udo Erasmus

COCONUT OIL MIRACLE OR MYTH? | 29

America. There are factors other than government nutritional guidelines that contribute to those statistics, but the change in our diet in the last 40+ years is the main culprit.

Anti-Saturated Fat Campaigns

The research studies that linked saturated fats with heart disease began as early as the 1850s[23] and took rise again in the 1950s by scientist and writer, Ancel Keys.

Keys concluded that saturated fats found in milk and meat were harmful and unsaturated fats found in vegetable oils were beneficial. This conclusion was based on an earlier hypothesis that all dietary fats cause obesity and cancer. We now know that obesity and cancer is largely caused by glucose (sugar).

Meanwhile, studies were carried out attributing an increased risk of coronary heart disease to elevated levels of serum cholesterol. Saturated fats and foods high in cholesterol were said to be the cause.

However, the link between saturated fats and serum cholesterol were never proven nor was the link between serum cholesterol and heart disease. Many scientists state that those links are frail at best. And yet this is the 'truth' we have all come to believe.

More recent studies (1991-) are taking the lead and dispelling the myth. It will take another 20 years before the results are shared and become common knowledge.

In any case, when all saturated fats were tossed in the bad-for-you pile, coconut oil went along for the ride. This was in err as you already know from reading the chapter titled "Coconut Oil's Fatty Acids". Even though the oil is classified as saturated, it doesn't act like saturated fat in the human body.

---

23 "Lipid hypothesis" http://en.wikipedia.org/wiki/Lipid_hypothesis

A widely believed conspiracy theory has founding in studies originating in the 1950s. A quote from the Weston A. Price Foundation's website is worthy of contemplation:

"...at that time (1960s) the edible oil industry in the United States seized the opportunity to promote its polyunsaturates. The industry did this by developing a health issue focusing on Key's anti-saturated fat bias. With the help of the edible oil industry lobbying in the United States, federal government dietary goals and guidelines were adopted incorporating this mistaken idea that consumption of saturated fat was causing heart disease. This anti-saturated fat issue became the agenda of government and private agencies in the US and to an extent in other parts of the world."[24]

The American Journal of Public Health[25] stated:

"...the focus of dietary recommendations is usually a reduction of saturated fat intake, no relation between saturated fat intake and risk of CHD was observed in the most informative prospective study to date."

Another quote is from William P. Castelli in the Archives of Internal Medicine (1992):

"...in Framingham, Mass, the more saturated fat one ate, the more cholesterol one ate, the more calories one ate, the lower the person's serum cholesterol...the opposite of what the equations provided by Hegsted at al (1965) and Keys et al (1957) would predict..."

The big takeaway on these reports conflicting with government nutrition guidelines is that five (or 50, or 100) research studies aren't enough.

---

24 "A New Look at Coconut Oil" by Mary G. Enig, PhD, 2000, http://www.westonaprice.org/know-your-fats/new-look-at-coconut-oil

25 "American Journal of Public Health", 1990, American Public Health Association, pg 1295

You must take personal responsibility for your own health. Do not allow it to slip into government's hands or rest upon scientist's shoulders.

Observe labels such as "health-smart" or "approved by the FDA" with a little less trust.

Eat a diet of natural and whole foods and leave any processed and pre-packaged food items (no matter what type of fats they contain) on the shelf.

I know this is a tall order.

Your longevity depends on it. You've already taken an interest in the wonderful benefits of coconut oil for your health, please continue on your quest of how simple and natural foods nourish you into a long and health-filled life.

Want to know more about the fat controversy and route we've taken to kill ourselves slowly?

Read "The Oiling of America", available free at: http://westonaprice.org/know-your-fats/the-oiling-of-america

[6]

INCORPORATING COCONUT OIL INTO YOUR LIFE

Coconut oil is an edible oil pressed from the kernel or meat of a coconut. The oil is available for sale at health food, grocery, and drug stores. You are likely to find it with cooking oils, or in the international cooking aisle of your grocery store. You might also see it with hair care products but this is not the oil you will want for the best results.

The oil is sold in glass bottles, plastic jars and economy-sized tubs. As it is a product of tropical countries its natural state is liquid. In North America where ambient room temperatures are at or below 76 degrees Fahrenheit, the oil is a solid.

Natural coconut oil has a shelf life of approximately two years post-packaging. Expiry dates should be printed on any coconut oil you purchase for consumption.

At home, you do not need to store coconut oil in the refrigerator. Let it sit on your counter and you'll use it more often. Opaque packaging protects the oil from the sun's rays. Reasonable variances in temperature won't affect quality. Coconuts are grown in the tropics – moderate heat won't alter the composition.

Choosing A Good Coconut Oil

Purchase the best quality you can afford. On average I spend about $12 per pound ($17 litre) making a special order from my small town health food store. While this seems a high price for cooking oil, once you know all the benefits, you won't mind the cost.

Prices have fluctuated over the years and they are on the rise to match market demand. Recent increases are largely due to the Paleo diet's popularity and Dr. Oz's[26] coverage on the benefits of coconut oil.

I estimate my cost at a dollar per day. Costs can be reduced by purchasing in bulk or ordering directly from the manufacturer. Shop first to find an oil you like, from a company with ethical harvesting and processing practices, before buying large tubs.

Not all coconut oil is created equal. Up until a few years ago the market was largely unregulated. Today, most companies share their harvesting and processing techniques online, some with photo proof. Online bloggers and health advocates voraciously share their favorite brands – which may help your research. Somewhere between the sales pitch and the research you'll find a company that suits your ethics. I would suggest a few brands myself, but business owners and harvesting practices are known to change – a printed word cannot.

What's On The Label?

Labels can be confusing and some are downright redundant. Many classifications are little more than justification for a higher price – especially so for the uninformed consumer.

---

26 A Turkish-American cardiothoracic surgeon and popular television personality.

Virgin, extra virgin, refined, unrefined, organic, non-GMO, pure, raw, cold pressed, expeller-pressed, centrifuged, hexane-free, non-bleached, zero trans fat, and zero hydrogenated fat are but a few of the distinctions.

Non-GMO & Certified Organic

As non-GMO (Genetically Modified Organism) is the biggest buzzword in health-conscious communities, let's start here. I fully support the decision to purchase non-GMO foods but when it comes to coconuts and coconut oil, this has no bearing on my selection.

My top 3 reasons why:

1. Many fine producers get their supply of coconuts from small farms and communities. Those coconuts are growing naturally, may be hybrid coconut palms, but aren't likely to be GMO.

2. Calls to action requesting the scientific community to create a GMO coconut palm[27] exist but to date none worthy of concern. I have yet to see evidence that GMO coconuts or products are in service, much less reaching North American shores.

3. The top 5 countries growing and producing coconut products have a natural, ample supply to meet current market demand. These are, in order of production: Indonesia, Philippines, India, Brazil, Sri Lanka.

As for a certified organic label, when the difference is just a few dollars more I'm happy to spend it. Companies that have taken the time, trouble and expense of organic certification are generally

---

27 "Develop genetically modified coconut, Pinoy scientists urged", (2009), http://www.philstar.com/science-and-technology/499275/develop-genetically-modified-coconut-pinoy-scientists-urged

quite passionate about their product. The coconuts would be grown, harvested, and processed by best industry practices.

However, during years of tight household budgets, I have dismissed the certification if the oil was labeled chemical-free or cold-pressed.

As this appears contradictory to my values, allow me to explain.

I'm more concerned about the extraction practice than I am about the growing practice.

Why?

Two reasons:

1. The chance of coconuts harvested in mass quantities from a polluted environment of fertilizers and pesticides is slim. Even if pesticides have been used, coconuts have a fairly resilient husk.

2. Some companies use harmful chemicals to dry or extract oil from coconut meat. It is enough for me to know that the oil was produced without the use of chemicals.

Should you need extra surety, The Environmental Working Group (a group of researchers in the United States) regularly test and list common foods for chemical and pesticide residue. Over the years coconut has been on the list of "Foods Less Likely To Be Tainted".[28]

Where the choices get difficult is in the difference between refined and unrefined.

---

28 If you're interested, you can stay updated from their website here: http://www.ewg.org/foodnews/

Refined vs. Unrefined Coconut Oil

When we look at all natural health food, we snub our noses at anything refined. Much like vegetables, all the healthful qualities can be cooked right out of a food, so raw is always best, right?

Research provides a different view.

Both refined and unrefined have benefits. Refined – even at high heat during processing – presents with a higher anti-oxidant count in some laboratory tests.[29]

If your interest lies mainly in the anti-oxidant qualities of coconut oil, refined may be the oil of choice.

Also, coconut oil (unless it is hydrogenated) still maintains medium chain fatty acid composition during refinement and high heat. This includes lauric acid – and the resulting monolaurin.

Refining is also an ancient tradition of processing coconuts.

With that said, there are some caveats about buying and using refined coconut oil:

1. Some companies refine and extract with chemicals. Look for organic or chemical-free on the label.

2. Some start with copra (dried coconut meat) that might not be of the highest quality. It is very hard to tell whether oil is made from quality copra or sub-standard copra when the oil has been refined. Research the company.

3. Should the label say RBD (refined, bleached and deodorized) the chemical processing is too high to risk. This oil has no value to health or beauty.

---

29 "Comparison of the phenolic-dependent antioxidant properties of coconut oil extracted under cold and hot conditions" (2008), in vitro and in vivo, http://wideliaikaputri.lecture.ub.ac.id/files/2012/09/11.-Comparison-of-the-phenolic-dependent-antioxidant-properties-of-coconut-oil.pdf

4. A refined oil, even when certified organic, can be less than ideal. In a 1974 book titled "Food For Naught: The Decline in Nutrition", author Dr. Ross Hall confirmed that coconut oil can become damaged when refined at temperatures just below its smoke point. Virgin coconut oil's smoke point is 350°F/177°C.

Virgin vs. Extra Virgin Coconut Oil

Coconut oil does not follow the same standards as olive oil in regards to virgin or extra virgin labeling.

The Asian and Pacific Coconut Community (APCC) standards state that "Virgin coconut oil is obtained from the fresh and mature kernel of coconut by mechanical or natural means with or without the application of heat, which does not lead to alteration of the oil."[30]

From that statement you can assume that a virgin label will protect the product from excessive heat. I'll assume that such a statement also implies chemical-free, but you will want to make your own assumptions.

Note that Brazil is the world's 4th largest producer of coconuts and not a member of the APCC. If the coconut oil in your cupboard is from Brazil, different standards may apply.

At the time of writing, no standard has been declared for extra virgin coconut oil although it has been showing up on labels.

Why? In olive oils the extra virgin label is allowed only when all criteria have been met:

- chemical free extraction,
- extraction within 24 hours of harvest,

30 APPC Standards for Virgin Coconut Oil,
http://www.apccsec.org/document/vcno.pdf

- first press only,
- cold press,
- and level of acidity.

Does the extra virgin label on jars of coconut oil signify a higher standard oil or is it just a dupe for a higher price?

Understanding Extraction Methods

Extraction methods include wet-milled, cold-pressed, centrifuged, or expeller-pressed. Wet-milled and expeller-pressed are similar methods that may use heat. Cold-pressed and centrifuged might also be subjected to heat, but temperatures are better controlled.

After the first extraction method, the liquid will be separated from the mash. Refrigeration, boiling, fermentation, the addition of enzymes, or any combination thereof will separate the oil from the liquid. The method chosen determines whether the oil will be labeled refined or unrefined.

Hexane-Free

Generally ignored by the marketplace, hexane-free is a worthy descriptive. I have yet to see the distinction make an impact on price even though I love to see it on my jars.

The use of hexane to extract oil from nuts and seeds is a long-standing and conventional practice. Very little, if any at all, hexane can be found in a finished oil. Hexane is a chemical solvent that can be dangerous to factory staff and to our environment over the long term.

Coconut Oils To Avoid

Aside from RBD (above) you'll also want to turn away from hydrogenated, partially hydrogenated, and/or fractionated oils.

Fractionated coconut oil – also labelled as liquid coconut oil – has the most beneficial component (lauric acid) stripped from it. These may seem to be a good deal or easier to cook with but leave them all on the shelf as the most certainly will do your body more harm than good.

What Is Coconut Butter?

People often confuse coconut butter with coconut oil. Coconut butter is cheap to buy but only contains 20-30% oil at best. This product is finely ground coconut meat with some liquid removed and is a nice addition to recipes in Eastern cuisine. Ounce for ounce it does not provide the same benefits as coconut oil.

Which Will You Choose?

Now that you know the many varieties which will you choose?

My suggestion, if your budget allows, is to shop first for organic or chemical-free. Next look for virgin or extra-virgin (if you know the manufacturing process).

Any of the extraction methods are fine when you have a virgin label, but the cold-pressed distinction is nice to see.

Stay away from refined until you've had a chance to research a company's extraction process, value system, and business ethics.

Learning Forward To Good Health

Good health, consistent energy levels, a clear and positive mind. These are the spoken promises in every article and book on coconut oil. Some go as far as calling it a miracle cure to the life-threatening diseases of modern man.

As much as I believe in the virtues of this simple oil I could never make such generalizations in person or in print.

I respect and am mindful of your personal health concerns.

You will find references to many ills in the following chapters. They have been – to the best of my ability – linked to research studies that support each theory or claim.

Should you have a serious illness - any illness - I urge you to continue your research long after you've read the last page of this book. Do so with a critical and skeptical mind.

Articles on websites are often little more than personal opinion subtly veiled with the intention of a sale. This slick marketing may read as though it was written from the heart but it is the commission, not your cure, that is the intent. Be a gatherer of facts – not a victim of hype.

Please talk to your doctor. Find a certified naturopath or nutritionist. Pick up a book on Aruyvedic or alternative health.

To find current research on any health concerns you may have, run a few searches on PubMed.com or any other reputable health sciences website. Search for studies on symptoms or diseases that concern or affect you. In search phrases be sure to specifically add "coconut oil", "medium-chain triglycerides", "lauric acid", "monolaurin", or "ketones" for best results.[31]

Coconut Oil In Your Diet

In the meantime, start using coconut oil daily. Notice how you feel throughout the day or how your skin feels when you use it as a moisturizer. Try it for a few weeks and then assess the changes in your appearance, energy level, and well being. It is wise practice to keep a health journal; recording how you feel each day while your body and skin adjust to this new addition.

---

31 If you would like to include an interesting study for future editions of this book, please contact the publisher.

If you're in good health, begin by taking one teaspoon per day. Slowly increase your intake over the course of the week to 3-4 teaspoons per day. This will cause the least digestive upset – should you experience any.

Three to four servings throughout the day is the recommended standard in clinical trials.

There are no published side effects to the ingestion of coconut oil when taken in moderation. Should you feel nauseous through the introduction phase, you might have a sensitivity to MCTs. This usually passes as your body adjusts. Reduce your intake or stop for a few weeks and try again.

You may be advised by others to take up to 4 tablespoons daily. I would suggest only doing so if you are fighting an infection or trying to lose weight.

If you are trying to lose weight, don't just add coconut oil, use it as a replacement of other oils in your diet. Swap out any other oil except for olive oil – the Omega 3s in olive oil are important to good health.

If you desire to take coconut oil only as preventative medicine, I don't believe any harm would come of taking 4 tablespoons daily.

Four tablespoons per day is the adult equivalent percentage of MCTs and lauric acid to that of a newborn baby drinking breast milk.

If you are a coffee drinker, try adding a ¼ teaspoon to your morning coffee. It will soften your lips while you drink it. Even if you find the idea repulsive, try it just once. You might notice a difference in energy and clarity during the first few hours of your day.

If you like smoothies or green drinks for breakfast, slowly add a teaspoon of warmed coconut oil to the blender while mixing.

Should your energy level crash mid-afternoon, take a teaspoon straight out of the jar. Within 10 minutes you will have forgotten about picking up that unhealthy snack for the commute – ample time to get home and cook a nutritious dinner.

As for snacks, you can pop corn in coconut oil and it can also replace the buttery topping.

Spread it on a slice of toast.

Freeze teaspoonfuls of it. Coconut oil is delicious frozen! Frozen fat doesn't sound delicious, but try it, at least once.

Roasted kale chips are a guilt-free snack when made with coconut oil.

Mix it into morning oatmeal; you won't notice a difference in taste or consistency.

Fry eggs in it; you will need half as much coconut oil as any other fat to keep your eggs from sticking to the pan.

Saute vegetables.

Replace butter or lard in nearly every baking recipe.

You're sure to find many more ways to incorporate it into your diet once you discover how versatile it is.

Coconut Oil For Self Care

Coconut oil is already in your bathroom cabinets. It is an industry-standard, base ingredient for soaps and shampoos.

Start using coconut oil as a face moisturizer and body lotion. Through repeated use the oil's antioxidant properties removes surface toxins from your skin while protecting it for the remainder of the day.

Perform A Patch Test

Have you ever done a patch test to test for a skin allergy? Here's a sensible 24 hour approach.

1. After a shower or bath, rub a little coconut oil onto the underside of your forearm; about 2" in diameter. Allow it to soak in for 10-20 minutes before getting dressed.

2. Over the next 24 hours, be aware of any sign of irritation - an annoying itch, redness, bumps, hives or swelling.

Give the detox process a kick start by taking a long, hot soak with 2 cups of epsom salts. Rinse off, moisturize with coconut oil, and you are on your way to a nourished glow!

Pick up some small, wide-mouthed, glass jars at a craft store or dollar store and fill them with your coconut oil. Place those jars in your path and you'll be more likely to use them. Take one to the office, leave one by your bedside, or your coffee table.

Every time you see one of those jars, use it. Rub some into your cuticles, on dry elbows. Put a little on your lips.

Men, don't balk, you can do this too! We all get chapped hands and lips.

Coconut Oil For Animal Care

Always check with your veterinarian before making changes to your pet's diet, especially if your pet has outstanding health concerns. I have never heard of a dog or cat having trouble digesting coconut oil but that doesn't mean it never happens.

Topically, coconut oil helps to:

- alleviate itchy or hot spots
- disinfect and promote healing of cuts, wounds or scrapes
- moisturize dry, itchy skin from contact allergies, flea allergies or eczema
- prevent and/or treat fungal infections
- remove dried fecal matter from long haired cats and dogs
- reduce burning, swelling or itching from insect stings

Internally, coconut oil may:

- aid in digestion
- help to eliminate hairballs
- increase energy and metabolism
- assist with arthritis
- improve nutrient and vitamin absorption
- prevent or control pet diabetes
- prevent infection and/or infectious disease

Start with a low dose and watch for changes in bowel movements, skin tone, energy levels and coat health.

The recommended dose for cats or dogs is ½ teaspoon per 10 pounds of body weight. Pets will eat it from their bowl, from your hand, or mixed into their food or water.

You should notice a change in your pet's energy level within a few days, coat within a week, and nails within 3 weeks. We have a terrier breed that is prone to the painful splintering of nails. In the last 2 years we haven't had one occurrence.

For years on the farm we also used coconut oil topically on horses, cows and goats. We would mix up a fresh jar every Spring adding a few drops of citronella essential oils per cup of coconut oil. Spread lightly, daily, on the inner and outer ear alleviated the itch of bug bites and seemed to discourage excessive bites.

Cows and goats received an udder rub of pure coconut oil every other day when dry; daily when lactating or feeding young. We lived 15 years free of mastitis and I give all the credit to coconut oil.

[7]

WHOLE BODY HEALTH & WELLNESS

This section deals with the benefits of coconut oil based on parts of, and functions of, our body. It includes both internal and external use.

Detox

Never has there been a era where it is necessary to detox our organs and systems than the one we're living in right now. Chemical toxins are in the air around us, they are in our food supply (even when we're eating properly), our water supply, and in our personal care products.

When a few toxins enter our system, our body usually flushes them out with the rest of the waste. If those toxins don't get flushed out, they turn into free radicals where they can accumulate, duplicate, and cause organ failure and cancer.

There are many ways to help your body flush out those toxins. Eating anti-oxidant rich foods, drinking alkaline water, or purchasing herbal kits are three of the most common methods.

Regular use of coconut oil will also help keep your system clean as well. It's anti-microbial properties keep your body balanced while supporting natural metabolic functions to flush out the toxins.

Ears, Eyes & Nose

Most of us spend 16 hours or more indoors with either the heat blowing or air conditioning blasting. In both instances moisture is removed from the air causing eyes, nostrils, and the surrounding skin to become itchy and irritated.

Virgin, organic coconut oil is a perfect lubricant to ease these irritations. The oil is as beneficial in your body as it is externally.

For dry, itchy eyes, lightly massage a small amount of oil around the surrounding skin. You can rub the oil directly onto your lashes and brows as it will not irritate your eyes but will nourish both hair and follicles (see the following chapter "Hair & Scalp").

For exceptionally itchy or dry eyes, place a few drops of slightly warmed (just to the point of liquid) coconut oil directly onto each eye. I didn't believe this could work – oil onto a saline-based organ – but it does. The lubricating and antibiotic properties work well together to combat irritations. Add the drops, close the eyelid, rest for about 2 minutes. Vision will be cloudy for about 30-45 seconds but your eyes will feel much better for the remainder of the day.

Treat an eye stye in the same manner as above by first washing the area gently, holding a warm compress to the area for 2-3 minutes and then adding in a few drops of coconut oil. Do this up to 3 times per day. Styes are usually caused by the Staphylococcus aureus bacterium which monolaurin has been proven to fight. In my experience this treatment shortens the duration of the sty. It may also prevent consecutive recurrences. Wash all towels, droppers, compresses and hands immediately after treatment.

Coconut oil can also be applied within nostrils. With head tilted back for 1-2 minutes, apply a few drops per nostril. This treatment – once every few days – has stopped my son's weekly nose bleeds for the last two winters. This may also help with chronic snoring.

Slight ear infections and itchy ears can be the result of a serious health problem that require a professional's care. Minor problems, when caught in time, are the result of a bacterial or fungal infection. Coconut oil's anti-microbial properties may alleviate symptoms or cure the problem altogether. See "Swimmer's Ear" (Chapter: A Long List of Cures) for more information.

Grooming

Have you read the label of your favorite shampoo or hand lotion? Nine times out of ten, one of the 10-30 items on the label will be a derivative of coconut oil. This has been the case for nearly a century.

Coconut oil makes an inexpensive base, products containing it are stable on the shelf for long periods of time, and consumers gets great results when using the products.

Some manufacturers, looking for better customer experiences, employ chemists to create cheaper, more stable products. To do so those chemists must alter what already exists in nature.

Trouble always follows.

The latest scandal – for lack of a better word - Cocomide DEA (a mixture of coconut oil and diethanolamine) has been identified as a likely carcinogenic. At the time of writing this book, nearly 200 popular shampoo and beauty products have been identified as containing the harmful compound.[32]

How ironic.

Coconut oil is a natural anti-oxidant and yet we smash it into some 3rd generation compound to create a product that could kill us. Then we spend $8 for the privilege of lathering our bodies in it.

Sadly, Cocomide DEA isn't an isolated incident. In 2010 Sodium Lauryl Sulfate (a compound partially made from coconut and palm oil) was found to be in thousands of shampoos and beauty products and was also thought to be carcinogenic.[33]

In the end it was considered "just an irritant" and continues to be used in the industry. There's more to this story than meets the eye and is yet another controversial conspiracy that few people have time to sift through.

Such things truly sadden me.

There are at least 30 compounds and derivatives of coconut oil used in the food and beauty industry. Most are well tested, safe, and have never caused a problem.

I thought I'd list them for you; then realized the futility. No sooner would this book be out then 5 new compounds would be approved for use.

Simplicity is best.

---

32 "Lawsuit Launched as Testing Finds Cancer-Causing Chemical in Nearly 100 Hair Care and Personal Care Products", August 2013, Center for Environmental Health http://www.ceh.org/news-events/press-releases/content/lawsuit-launched-testing-finds-cancer-causing-chemical-in-100-shampoos-haircare-products/

33 "Sodium Lauryl Sulfate Use in Cosmetics", March 2010, http://davidsuzuki.org/issues/health/science/toxics/chemicals-in-your-cosmetics---sodium-laureth-sulfate/

Natural is healthier.

You can enjoy the beauty benefits of coconut oil, without the harmful chemicals, and at a fraction of the price.

Want to know how?

"Just put some coconut oil on it!"

Virgin coconut oil is an all-natural, chemical and fragrance-free, quick absorbing, and non-greasy moisturizer.

It is perfect for use as a hand cream, face moisturizer, eye cream, body lotion, after shave, cuticle cream, foot lotion, hair mask and make up remover – no mixing or measuring required. Perfect for sensitive skin types.

Massage into, as often as required, freshly washed skin. If you have an acne break-out in the first week of use, this does not mean the oil is too greasy for your skin type. More often it is the oil's detoxification at work, clearing your skin of impurities.

It comes out of the jar ready to:

- soothe sunburns, bug bites, and hives
- protect open wounds and scrapes from dirt and bacteria
- heal chapped lips
- prevent razor burn
- remove make up
- kill viruses and bacteria
- treat eczema, dermatitis, psoriasis, and other skin problems; and
- alleviate symptoms of (sub type 1 and 2) rosacea and contact dermatitis.

With regular use it may also:

- detox skin's top layers
- minimize scars
- restore skin elasticity; and
- reduce the appearance of fine lines and wrinkles.

Age spots (solar lentigines or liver spots) are a common skin complaint. These spots are often found on the backs of hands, tops of feet, face and shoulders, on all skin types over 40+ years of age.

Age spots are not an indication of liver malfunction, but of sun exposure. The testimonials found online regarding the removal or reduction of age spots are without evidence nor supportive theory.

Hair & Scalp

Right out of the jar:

- control split ends
- increase shine and volume
- smooth static and frizz; and
- prevent and treat dandruff.

Prevent Dandruff

You have a fungus growing on your scalp.

Don't worry, everyone has it, even people without dandruff.

Hair follicles create oils that the malassezia fungi feed upon. When oil production is high, more malassezia grows. The overgrowth of fungi causes irritation and our scalp flakes. When oil production is low, a scalp will also flake.

Both types benefit from coconut oil. Coconut oil moisturizes dry scalp as well as combats fungi overgrowth.

Massage a teaspoon of slightly warmed coconut oil into scalp a few times per week. Leave on for 20 minutes or longer. Wash and style hair as usual.

Flyaway Hair and Split Ends

A coconut oil treatment helps to prevent static hair as well as seal split ends. While split ends cannot be 'cured' coconut oil will help them from worsening. If split ends are a common problem, be sure to give your hair a coconut oil treatment every week between haircuts.

Baldness, Receding Hairline and Thinning

"Rub some coconut oil on your scalp every day for a month and your hair will come back."

The "curing baldness" industry is almost as large as the weight loss industry. As such, it is rife with snake oil sales of all types.

Let's be real.

There are many causes for hair loss. Diet, stress, medications, environmental conditions, genetics, and hormonal changes are just a few of the reasons our hair thins, recedes, or stops growing altogether.

Can coconut oil help us balance some of those issues? It sure can, but that does not mean taking it, rubbing it on your scalp every day or any other cited technique will make hair grow again.

Rub it on your scalp to increase blood flow, moisturize the area, and keep (natural) scalp fungi balanced. You'll be creating a lovely environment that supports hair growth but isn't likely to promote hair growth.

If hormonal imbalances are the cause of hair loss, add coconut oil to your diet to support thyroid and adrenal glands. Hormones might stabilize, which could result in hair growth.

Pamper Thinning Hair

> "Among three oils, coconut oil was the only oil found to reduce the protein loss remarkably for both undamaged and damaged hair when used as a pre-wash and post-wash grooming product."[34]

Finally, pamper the hair you have left on your head by using a coconut hair mask once per week. Each hair absorbs and is coated by the coconut oil to protect it from the sun (SPF 4-6), from environmental toxins, and from repeated use of combs and styling appliances.

Immune System

There is great promise and research in the ways coconut oil supports our immune system. A strong immune system can fight off viruses and bacteria but can also battle and rid our system of mutant cells before they cause disease, cancers, or other system failures.

We all have the potential for cancer cells – or imperfect cell structure during a cell's life. Our immune system works to keep those cells in check by removing or preventing them from deviating further or reproducing.

Coconut oil packs a one-two punch to keep the immune system strong and, hopefully, cancer at bay.

Monolaurin, the by-product of lauric acid, has been proven to stimulate the production of T cells (white blood cells), which have

---

34 "Effect of mineral oil, sunflower oil, and coconut oil on prevention of hair damage." 2003 http://www.ncbi.nlm.nih.gov/pubmed/12715094

been proven to destroy cancerous cells. Medium-chain fatty acids have been shown to inhibit over-growth of tumors that have already started.[35]

Intestinal / Digestive Tract

Our intestinal and digestive tracts are loaded with good bacteria. They help to digest dairy products such as milk and cheese, convert foods into vitamins, and fight off bad bacteria, viruses and yeasts that we come into contact with.

Problems associated with the digestive tract are caused by an imbalance between good and bad bacteria; or virus and yeast organisms multiplying past the point of a healthful balance. Digestive troubles can show up as a variety of symptoms – from acne to allergies, indigestion to ulcers.

Coconut oil's anti-microbial properties selectively attack and nullify harmful organisms and restore balance to the digestive tract.

Liver

The liver is one of the hardest working organs in your body. It reconstructs the composition of fats and proteins and converts the end product to useful energy. The liver also stores excess fats and proteins for later use.

One of the liver's most important tasks is to filter out and neutralize toxins. As such, it takes the hardest hit. Coconut oil supports the liver by working in conjunction with it. The oil kills germs, neutralizes free radicals, and feeds the liver with lovely

---

35 "Integration of Metabolism, Energetics, and Signal Transduction: Unifying Foundations in Cell Growth and Death, Cancer, Atherosclerosis, and Alzheimer Disease" (specifically Chapter 4), 2004, Robert K. Ockner

MCFAs. This reduces stress on the liver, allowing more energy to be used for stimulating metabolic function.

Teeth and Gums

The ingestion of coconut oil will improve calcium and magnesium absorption – two beneficial minerals for dental and bone health. Improved calcium absorption has been proven to deter tooth decay.

As you already know, coconut oil is an anti-bacterial. Gum disease, gingivitis[36] , and bad breath are caused by bacteria.

Rubbing coconut oil directly on the gums twice daily, using a coconut-oil based toothpaste and following the ancient practice of oil-pulling maintains oral health.

If you've had dental work or oral surgery you can prevent the complications brought on by infection by gently rubbing coconut oil into the area twice daily. Doing so may also speed healing time. If you have stitches, practice gentle oil-pulling twice per day.

Thyroid

The thyroid gland regulates metabolism through a wide array of functions. A sluggish or damaged thyroid can cause problems with digestion, immune system response, the speed at which you heal, and the speed of hormone and enzyme production.

36 "Effect of oil pulling on plaque induced gingivitis: a randomized, controlled, triple-blind study.", 2009, http://www.ncbi.nlm.nih.gov/pubmed/19336860

Abnormal changes in body function that aren't easily explained are often a sign of thyroid trouble.

Symptoms of a damaged thyroid are:

- constipation
- depression
- hypoglycemia
- insomnia
- joint pain
- migraines; and
- yeast infections

Coconut oil's MCFAs help to alleviate symptoms of a damaged thyroid. When the cause of a sluggish or damaged thyroid is dietary or induced by stress, regular use of coconut oil supports and may repair the metabolic functions of the thyroid.

Oil Pulling Therapy

An Ayurvedic practice considered to cure 30 systemic diseases. Traditionally performed with sesame oil.

Swish 1/2 teaspoon of oil through the mouth for 4-6 minutes and expel. As you 'swish', pull the oil through the teeth, from cheek to cheek, under your tongue, and behind your back molars.

A study using sesame oil (which does not have the anti-microbial qualities of coconut oil) shows a statistically significant reduction of plaque and gingival index scores.

Women's Health

Women may have more to gain from the use of coconut oil then men – simply due to hormonal changes and pregnancy.

Using virgin coconut oil as a daily moisturizer may prevent or reduce the appearance of stretch marks. It also conditions and protect the perineum for and during childbirth.

Medicinally, the oil provides the same benefits to a woman as it does to her unborn child, the least of which is a stronger immunity. Coconut oil has also been used to treat morning sickness and may be beneficial in the prevention of gestational diabetes due to maintaining healthy and stable blood glucose levels.

When a breastfeeding mother ingests coconut oil, the fatty acid composition in her milk changes. The largest increase occurs within the first 14 hours but can continue up to 3 days.[37]

In North America, lauric acid makes up about 6% of the saturated fats in breast milk. Lauric acid content has been recorded as high as 15% in countries where coconut is a dietary staple.

Cracked nipples and mastitis are painful and potential complications in breastfeeding. Coconut oil's anti-bacterial properties – applied topically and ingested, help to prevent both.

In later years, coconut oil may also help prevent osteoporosis. Scientists currently believe that osteoporosis could be caused by unbalanced levels of progesterone and estrogen. During menopause, when estrogen levels are high, extra progesterone could be beneficial. One of coconut oil's sterols is structurally

---

37 "Acute effects of dietary fatty acids on the fatty acids of human milk.", 1998, http://ajcn.nutrition.org/content/67/2/301.abstract

similar to pregnenolone which converts to progesterone when consumed.

Weight & Fitness

According to scientists at McGill University in Montreal Canada, diets high in MCFAs increase metabolism.

The McGill study reviewed over 30 previous research reports and ascertained that if the average person made no other changes to their lifestyle but to replace current dietary fats with virgin coconut oil, he/she could lose up to 35 pounds in the first year.

The study was so successful that Forbes Medi-Tech and the Dairy Farmers of Canada commissioned a further study at the cost of $400,000. The result of the second study was a formulation that created a better dietary oil comprised of 71% tropical and coconut oils.[38]

With this knowledge of coconut oil and your metabolism, plus what you've already learned in this book about how our bodies use MCFAs, you can see the power of using coconut oil to lose weight. Not only does the oil provide energy and nourishment, support multiple bodily functions, but it also tastes great and is easy to cook with.

Here are four quick facts about coconut oil and weight loss:

1. The biggest metabolic boost occurs within the first 2 hours of ingestion, but continues for up to 24 hours.
2. Suppresses appetite by immediately feeding your body.
3. Decreases cravings by providing quick energy.
4. Does not store as body fat.

---

38 "Fat-fighting functional oil" (2003),
   http://www.mcgill.ca/reporter/35/16/jones/

If you are considering coconut oil for weight loss, or any of the high-fat, low-carb diets I've discussed within these pages, it is important to know more about dietary fats and what happens when we consume them.

From the earlier chapter on fats you already know the difference between some fats and oil, saturated and unsaturated and hydrogenation. I'm also assuming that you know you need a balance of fats that should also include sources of omega-3 and omega-6 fats.

Are You Tired In The Afternoon?

If you suffer from afternoon lows (the most probable time to reach for an unhealthy snack), take a teaspoon of coconut oil. It will boost your metabolism, clear brain fog, and satisfy your hunger for at least 2 hours.

While the McGill study may state that switching all fats over to virgin coconut oil results in weight loss, it isn't the healthiest way for your body to lose weight.

Long-chain fatty acids have a tendency to stick together which is why too much of this fat, makes us fat. We need LCFAs because they are required to build cell membranes.

Medium-chain fatty acids, as you know, are used as energy and not stored as body fat.

Then, there is the fatty acids our bodies create. When we eat too much refined sugar and starch, our pancreas secretes insulin. Insulin carries the excess to our cells. If our cells don't use the excess, our body starts converting the excess sugar and starch to fat. When 3 fatty acids connect to a glycerol molecule, a new molecule is formed. A fat molecule. That new fat molecule is then sent into the bloodstream looking for a place to settle until it is needed - if it is needed.

Finally, even though our bodies can create fatty acids from excess sugar and starch to use as energy, this process is unnecessary. We get all the fatty acids our bodies require for energy and cell regeneration from natural fats contained in real food.

In conclusion, if you are looking at coconut oil as a means to lose weight, it would behoove you to research a low-carb, high fat diet and replace only part of (not all) your dietary or cooking fat with coconut oil.

[8]

AILMENTS & DISEASE

Modern Medications - *Antibiotics work for most bacterial infections but they will not kill a virus. Most viruses will run their course. As long as your immune system is strong, you'll get well.*

Antiviral medications are not capable of killing the virus, but they will reduce the viral load while your body does the lion's share of the work.

Vaccines prevent serious viral diseases. Modern medicine does so by introducing the virus to our body. Our bodies react by triggering our immune system to create antibodies.

Coconut oil's natural anti-viral, anti-inflammatory, anti-bacterial and anti-fungal properties make it an excellent topical treatment for everything from acne to toenail fungus. Some of the ailments below might have more than one contributing factor which will determine your success of using coconut oil as a treatment.

Taken internally, coconut oil is believed to help, prevent, or alleviate the symptoms of the following health problems and illnesses.

Some have extensive research studies to back the claims. Others have been used in Aruyvedic medicine for centuries. Some are realistic once you've read this book and understand the properties and composition of coconut oil. Others are deserving of a raised eyebrow only.

Lists like the one below can be found on multiple websites and may be more extensive. Extensive, but seldom researched for validity, seldom challenged. Please consult with a naturopathic or other medical professional, and perform extensive and reputable research for any claim.

As an example (and this may not apply specifically to your case), coconut oil is being touted as helpful for Acid Reflux. The truth is that some sufferers have problems digesting any type of fat due to gallbladder or liver problems. While coconut oil isn't likely to cause damage, it might exacerbate the symptoms of Acid Reflux.

As with any physical ailment and a treatment - certainly before putting all your faith in coconut oil as a treatment of choice - observe the cause. Here's an example of this point: Carpal Tunnel Syndrome might be a sign of thyroid malfunction. It might also be caused by repetitive work stress. So while coconut oil is said to support thyroid functions, it does not alleviate the pain and suffering of cashiers and data entry clerks.

Determine the cause. Do your research. And never trust a list on your computer monitor - even mine.

With all those caveats out of the way I hope the list below intrigues and inspires you to seek out new knowledge – even those that appear to be on the edge of reason. For personal reasons I became very interested in coconut oil's effect on dementia patients. At a tertiary glance this seems preposterous, but logical reasoning based on coconut oil's composition; paired with multiple ongoing studies (some with wonderful results) has made me think twice.

Understanding The Chart

If you have read from the start of this book the following note style will be easy to follow as you now have discernment. Here you will put into practice all that you have learned.

I have scoured books and websites compiling a list of illnesses and diseases that others claim to cure with coconut oil. You will also find an updates and errata page at hulabooks.com/coconut-oil-errata/.

While coconut oil's use for some of the following ailments seem straight forward, more serious diseases will require a leap of faith. Those have been included based on research and theory. When possible, I note the theory(s).

Every item should be considered alternative medicine or a home remedy. Where a note states "usually treated by antibiotics," see a doctor.

Pregnant or lactating women, and children should always consult their medical practitioner.

For life-threatening diseases, please be sure to read later chapters – specifically "Research & Promises".

Topical: Apply topically as often as needed. Perform a patch test and wait 24 hours for a reaction before prolonged use.

Dietary / Preventative: Take coconut oil as a dietary supplement or replace a substantial percentage of your current cooking oil with coconut oil (up to 4 tablespoons daily).

Dietary / Medicinal: Prescribed usage varies. See the following section titled: "How Much Should I Take?" for direction.

Long List of Cures

Acne / Acne Vulgaris / Inflammatory Acne

When caused by bacteria.
Lauric and capric acid's anti-microbial qualities.
Dietary – to support immune system.
Topical – twice daily on freshly washed skin, reapply as needed.

Adrenal Fatigue / Adrenal Failure

Lauric acid supports hormonal functions of adrenal glands.
Dietary / Preventative.

ADHD

See Attention Deficit Disorder.

Alzheimer's & Dementia

A progressive disease of the brain.
Speculations on cause is varied.
Theory: (1) Said to be irreversible, but personal testimonies state improvement and/or slowed degeneration.[39]
(2) Coconut oil ingestion leads to an increase in blood ketones; directly affecting brain metabolism.
See Chapter: Research & Promises, specifically Neurological & Degenerative Diseases and Disorders
Dietary / Preventative.
Medicinal – to slow degeneration (anecdotal).

Amyotrophic lateral sclerosis (ALS)

ALS is a motor neuron disease without a cure. Speculations on the cause are varied and inconclusive.
See Chapter: Research & Promises, specifically Neurological & Degenerative Diseases and Disorders
Dietary / Preventative.
Medicinal – to slow degeneration (anecdotal).

---

39 "Alzheimer's Disease: What If There Was a Cure?" (2011) Mary T. Newport, http://www.amazon.com/Alzheimers-Disease-What-There-Cure/dp/1591202930

Animal & Snake Bites

Prevents infection and promotes healing. In minor bites it may relieve some pain or burning sensation.
Might neutralize some snake venom.
Always see a doctor and/or contact your local Animal Control authority.
Topical - immediately and hourly.

Anxiety

See Depression.

Asthma

Alleviates symptoms when asthma is caused by candida or diet.
Dietary / Preventative.
Medicinal – (see Candida albicans).

Athletes Foot

Fungal infection. Anti-fungal properties of coconut oil.
Topical – 2-3 times daily or as required.

Attention Deficit Disorder

The cause of ADD/ADHD has not yet been determined.
Speculations abound regarding genetics, diet, environmental, allergies, intestinal, and neural.
Studies are in progress.
When intestinal or neural is thought to be the cause, coconut oil (Essential Fatty Acids, fish oils) is common in alternative medicine trials.
Dietary / Medicinal.

Autism

A neural development disorder.
Theory: (1) Coconut oil ingestion leads to an increase in blood ketones; directly affecting brain metabolism.
(2) Vitamin D deficiencies in mother during pregnancy and toddler could be a contributing factor. Coconut oil assists in better Vitamin D absorption.
Studies are in progress.[40]
See Chapter: Research & Promises, specifically Neurological & Degenerative Diseases and Disorders.
Dietary / Medicinal.

Avian Flu

See Lipid-Coated Virus.

Bad Breath / Halitosis

When caused by bacteria.
See chapter: Whole Body Health & Wellness, specifically Teeth and Gums
Oral – twice daily.

Bed Sores / Pressure Ulcers

Relieves symptoms, prevents infection, and facilitates healing of stage 1 and 2 ulcers and sores.
Topical – 3-4 times daily or as required.

Benign Prostatic Hyperplasia

See Prostate Enlargement.

Bladder Infection

See Cystitis.

---

40 "Immunological and autoimmune considerations of Autism Spectrum Disorders." (2013) http://www.ncbi.nlm.nih.gov/pubmed/23867105

Blood Pressure Regulation

Anti-oxidants reduce oxidative stress and support heart function.
Dietary.

Boils / Cysts

When caused by compromised immune system or bacterial
infection.
Dietary to support immune system.
Topical as an anti-bacterial – twice daily on clean skin, reapply as
necessary.

Broken Bones

Supports the healing process, and possibly future breaks when
taken with (fat-soluble) Vitamin D and calcium supplements.
Dietary – with supplements.

Bronchial Infections / Acute Bronchitis (not Chronic)

When caused by virus or bacteria, usually follows a cold. See
Lipid-Coated Virus, Lipid-Coated Bacteria.
Dietary / Preventative – for immunity.
Medicinal when caused by virus or bacteria.

Cancer

Theory: Anti-microbial properties (monolaurin) of coconut oil is
said to prevent the spread of some cancer cells and support the
immune system.
See Chapter: Research & Promises, specifically Cancer.
Dietary / Medicinal – health management.
Dietary / Preventative (perhaps).[41]

---

41 "Effect of dietary fat saturation on survival of mice with L1210 leukemia."
   (1978) http://www.ncbi.nlm.nih.gov/pubmed/277734

Candida Albicans Infection

Fungal infection.
Capric and lauric acid have been proven to kill over proliferation of candida albicans.[42]
Topical / Medicinal
For vaginal infection, – ½ teaspoon of coconut oil frozen in a vaginal suppository shape at bedtime.
For throat infection (Thrush), gargle ½ teaspoon deeply and expel, 4 times per day.

Canker Sores

When caused by impaired immune system.
Dietary / Preventative.

Carpal Tunnel Syndrome

When it presents as a symptom of adrenal/thyroid malfunction.
See Adrenal Fatigue.

Cataracts

When caused by oxidative stress (e.g. aging).
Dietary / Preventative.

Celiac Disease

See Digestive Disorder.

Chicken Pox

Highly contagious viral disease. Vaccine is available. No known cure. Coconut oil relieves itching and reduces inflammation.
Dietary / Preventative – to support immunity.
Topical – to ease symptoms.

---

42 "In vitro killing of Candida albicans by fatty acids and monoglycerides."
     (2001) http://www.ncbi.nlm.nih.gov/pmc/articles/PMC90807/

Cholesterol Levels

Shown to improve the HDL (good cholesterol) to LDL ratio in multiple studies.
See Chapter: Composition of Coconut Oil, specifically Lauric Acid and Cholesterol

Chlamydia

Highly contagious sexually transmitted disease caused by the bacteria Chlamydia trachomatis.
Traditionally cured by antibiotics.
Capric acid and monocaprin have been shown to kill off Chlamydia trachomatis.[43]
Topical / Medicinal (alternative medicine).

Cold Sores / HSV-1

Anti-microbial component of monolaurin reduces the viral load.[44]

See Lipid-Coated Virus.
Dietary, Preventative – to keep immune strong and outbreaks minimal.
Topical – at first tingle of a cold sore and again to speed healing after first crack of the blister.

Common Cold

Viral infectious disease lasting 7-10 days. No cure.
Cold medications treat symptoms only.
See RSV.
Dietary / Preventative – to support immune system.

Conjunctivitis / Pink Eye

When caused by virus and/or bacteria.
Topical – apply along the eyelid or place a few drops directly onto the eye, twice daily.

---

43 "In vitro inactivation of Chlamydia trachomatis by fatty acids and monoglycerides." (1998) http://www.ncbi.nlm.nih.gov/pubmed/9736551

44 "Herpes" (2009), http://www.westonaprice.org/ask-the-doctor/herpes

Cradle Cap

Could be caused by a mild fungal infection. If it persists or if worsens a visit to the doctor is warranted.

Topical – rub a teaspoon of warmed coconut oil onto the cradle cap daily. Moisturizes, manages fungi and prevents any bacterial infection.

Crohn's Disease

See Digestive Disorder.

Croup

Usually a viral infection caused by the parainfluenza virus (flu) but can be further complicated by a bacterial virus. Usually clears itself in 48 hours.

Topical – two drops of eucalyptus essential oil (or lavender, or oregano) in a ¼ cup of warmed coconut oil rubbed on the back, chest and bottom of feet (alternative medicine).

Cystic Fibrosis

Coconut oil assists with some of the complications: pancreatic failure, bacterial infection in lungs, malabsorption of fat soluble vitamins, and constipation.

Dietary / Medicinal – (to prevent complications).

Cystitis / Urinary Tract Infection / Bladder Infection

Bacterial infection of urethra, ureter, bladder or kidneys. Most often caused by strains of Escherichia coli (E. coli is normal and natural gut flora). Usually treated by antibiotics but some strains are showing antibiotic resistance.

Dietary / Preventative.

Cytomegalovirus

See Lipid-Coated Virus.

Dementia

See Alzheimer's.

Depression

Increases blood ketone levels which directly affect and support brain function.
Dietary / Preventative - supportive.

Diabetes

Coconut oil provides nearly immediate energy to the body (much like a carbohydrate) without producing an insulin spike. Medium-chain fatty acids do not require pancreatic activity for absorption.
See Chapter: Research & Promises, specifically Diabetes.
Dietary / Medicinal – supportive only.

Diaper Rash

This rash has many causes. When it is mild or caused by a fungal (yeast) or bacterial infection, coconut oil both soothes and clears the rash.
Topical – apply at every diaper change to clean, dry skin.

Digestive Disorder

Digestive Disorders lead to a multitude of infections from micro-organisms - yeast, fungi, parasites, and viruses - as well as complications of the disorder including gastric ulcers, vitamin deficiency and a compromised immune system.
Anti-microbial and healing properties of coconut oil may address infections, symptoms and complications. Proceed with caution, not all sufferers react positively.
See Chapter: Research & Promises, specifically Irritable Bowel & Inflammatory Disease.
Dietary / Preventative – to support immune system.
Dietary / Medicinal – based on infection or complication.

Diverticulitis

See Digestive Disorder.

Dysentery

Dysentery can be caused caused by viral infection, bacterial infection, and parasitic infestation.
Dietary / Preventative.

Ear Infection (Acute Otitis Externa)[45]

A microbial infection that can clear on its own or with antibiotic ear drops. Coconut oil's antimicrobial qualities may clear mild cases.
Topical / Medicinal – as a home remedy. Two drops of slightly warmed oil inside the ear and resting for 5 minutes; twice daily for 2 days. If pain persists, see a professional. If infection is clearing, continue treatment for another 5 days.

Eczema

Alleviates symptoms (dryness, recurring rashes, redness, itching, crusting, flaking, blistering, cracking, oozing, or bleeding).
Supports immune system.
Topical - apply often.
Dietary / Preventative

Edema

When caused by adrenal malfunction or hormonal imbalance.
Dietary / Medicinal – supportive only.

Endometriosis

May help alleviate symptoms such as constipation and fatigue.

Epilepsy

Dietary change (saturated fat, low carb) puts the body into a starvation state (aka ketosis) which reduces the number and severity of seizures.
See Chapter: Research & Promises, specifically Neurological & Degenerative Diseases and Disorders

---

45 Does not include Otitis media or Labyrinthitis.

Epstein-Barr

See Lipid-Coated Virus.

Food Poisoning

When caused by bacteria.
Dietary / Medicinal - alternative medicine.

Gastritis / GERD

See Indigestion / Heartburn.

Giardiasis

Parasitic infection caused by the protozoan parasite Giardia lamblia. Lauric acid has been proven to kill giardia at rates comparable to the most prescribed medication.[46]
Dietary / Medicinal - alternative medicine.

Genital Herpes / HSV-2

Anti-microbial component of monolaurin reduces the viral load.
See Cold Sores / HSV-1 and Lipid-Coated Virus.
Dietary – preventative (to keep immune strong and outbreaks minimal).

Genital Warts (HPV)

See Warts.

Gonorrhea

A bacterial infection. Highly contagious with serious complications if left untreated.
In lab tests lauric and capric acids were both found to effectively kill gonorrhea bacteria.[47]
Dietary / Medicinal – alternative medicine.

---

46 "The effects of saturated fatty acids on Giardia duodenalis trophozoites in vitro." (2005) http://www.ncbi.nlm.nih.gov/pubmed/15991042

47 In Vitro Susceptibilities of Neisseria gonorrhoeae to Fatty Acids and Monoglycerides (1999) http://aac.asm.org/content/43/11/2790.full

Gout

Caused by high levels of uric acid in the body. When cause is dietary, coconut oil's ability to distribute magnesium help alleviate symptoms.
Dietary / Medicinal - 1 to 2 teaspoonfuls of coconut oil daily, along with vitamin E, magnesium and potassium supplements (alternative medicine).

Grave's Disease

An auto-immune disease that primarily affects the thyroid gland. Cause is unknown but thought to be genetic. Coconut oil supports thyroid function.
Dietary / Preventative – and proactive.

Gum Disease

See Chapter: Whole Health & Wellness, specifically Teeth & Gums.

Hang Nails

Used regularly will moisturize cuticles and area surrounding the nail bed to prevent hang nails. Hastens healing and prevents infection of existing hangnails.
Topical – apply often.

Hasimoto's / Thyroid Failure

May help alleviate symptoms such as fatigue, weight gain and constipation.
Dietary / Medicinal – supportive only.

Headache

When caused by stress.
Topical - rub coconut oil deep into the muscles between the thumb and pointer finger for 3-5 minutes (home remedy).

Heartburn

See Indigestion.

Helicobacter Pylori Infection

Helicobacter pylori is a bacterium found in the stomach that has been linked to chronic gastritis, gastric ulcers and stomach cancer.
See Lipid-Coated Bacteria.
Dietary / Medicinal – 1 teaspoon, 3 times daily, for 4 weeks (alternative medicine)[48] [49] .

Hepatitis C

Infectious viral disease usually attacking the liver. Coconut oil may reduce viral load.
Dietary / Preventative
Dietary / Medicinal – alternative medicine.

Herpes Simplex Virus

See Lipid-Coated Virus, Cold Sores, and/or Genital Herpes.

HPV

See Warts.

HSV-1

See Cold Sores.

HSV-2

See Genital Herpes.

Human Immunodeficiency Virus HIV-1, HIV+

Dietary / Medicinal – see Lipid-Coated Virus.

Human Respiratory Syncytial Virus

See RSV.

---

48 "Virgin Coconut Oil and Stomach Acid", Dr. Sanford Pinna, (2011), http://drpinna.com/virgin-coconut-oil-and-stomach-acid-16443

49 "Susceptibility of Helicobacter pylori to bactericidal properties of medium-chain monoglycerides and free fatty acids." (1996), http://www.ncbi.nlm.nih.gov/pmc/articles/PMC163106/

Human Lymphotropic (type 1)

See Lipid-Coated Virus.

Hyperthyroidism

See Grave's Disease.

IBS

See Digestive Disorder.

Impetigo

A highly contagious bacterial skin infection.
See Lipid-Coated Bacteria.
Topical – apply often.
Dietary / Medicinal – to support immune system.

Impotence

Coconut water is reported to boost blood circulation. Coconut oil is acclaimed by some to cure impotence. No research or logic can be found.
Dietary.

Indigestion

When caused by helicobacter pylori, auto-immune disorders, or bacterial infection.
Note: introduce coconut oil into your diet slowly. Discontinue use and talk to a health practitioner if problem persists.
Dietary[50] / Medicinal – alternative medicine. 1/2 teaspoon coconut oil with ¼ teaspoon cinnamon when affected.
Also see: Helicobacter Pylori.

Ingrown Hairs

Inhibits unnatural cell production and follicle plugs. May assist with puffiness of the area.
Topical – 3-5 times daily or as needed.

---

50 Conflicting evidence and testimonies. Suggestion: Introduce coconut oil into your diet slowly. Discontinue use if problem persists.

Influenza

See Lipid-Coated Virus.

Irritable Bowel Syndrome

See Digestive Disorder.

Jaundice

Commonly caused by liver or pancreas failure or disease.
Dietary / Preventative – supportive only.

Jock Itch

Anti-fungal properties reduce itch and burning sensation.
Topical – twice daily or as needed.

Keloids / Keartosis Pilaris[51]

See Ingrown Hairs.

Laryngitis

See Sore Throat.

Leaky Gut Syndrome

See Digestive Disorder.

Leg Cramps

See Muscle Cramps.

Leukemia

Cancer of the blood or bone marrow. Conventional medicine
doesn't always cure but can treat and manage symptoms.
Preliminary research on saturated fats and Leukemia have
extended life in rats.
See Chapter: Research & Promises, specifically Cancer.

---

51 Keloids - a collagen overgrowth often as a result of a scar. Keratosis pilaris –
an excess of protein of the skin.

Lipid-Coated Bacteria (LCB)

Monolaurin has been documented to attack and kill certain LCBs that cause illness and disease.
See Chapter: How Monolaurin Kills Lipid-Coated Viruses & Bacteria.
Dietary / Medicinal – alternative medicine.

Lipid-Coated Virus (LCV)

Monolaurin has been documented to attack and kill LCVs.
See Chapter: How Monolaurin Kills Lipid-Coated Viruses & Bacteria.
Dietary / Medicinal – alternative medicine.

Listeriosis

A bacterial infection most often caused by contaminated food.
See Lipid-Coated Bacteria.

Lou Gehrig's Disease

See Amyotrophic lateral sclerosis (ALS)

Lupus

May help with neurological and systemic conditions.
See Chapter: Research & Promises, specifically Autoimmune Disorders & Disease

Lyme Disease

Bacterial infection transmitted by a tick. Manifests as a circular spreading rash, 3-30 days after the tick bite. If caught in time this can be treated with one round of antibiotics. If not, the disease becomes difficult to treat and complications are so severe the disease can be described as a pathogen-induced autoimmune disease. Monolaurin supplements (as well as many other treatments) are used by some alternative health practitioners for advanced cases.
See Chapter: Research & Promises, specifically Auto-immune Disease.
Dietary / Medicinal – alternative medicine.

Measles / Measles Rubeola

Highly contagious viral disease of the respiratory system. Vaccination is available. Virus often runs it course in 5-7 days but complications can occur. Susceptibilities include Vitamin A deficiency, immunodeficiency, and malnutrition – all of which coconut oil prevents.
Dietary / Medicinal – see Lipid-Coated Virus.
Topical - to alleviate symptoms and prevent some complications.

Mononucleosis / Infectious mononucleosis (IM)

Infectious disease – most often caused by the Epstein-Barr virus but sometimes by Cytomegalovirus – both are lipid-coated and proven to be eradicated by Monolaurin.
In most cases Mononucleosis will run its course without symptoms or complications, however any discomfort should be discussed with a medical practitioner.
See Lipid-Coated Virus.

Mood Disorders

See Depression.

MRSA

See Staph Infection.

Muscle Cramps

When caused by a lack of calcium, potassium, and/or magnesium. Coconut oil assists with absorption of fat-soluble vitamins that work in harmony with these minerals.
Dietary / Preventative.

Nail Fungus

Anti-fungal properties of coconut oil relieve fingernail and toenail fungus.
Topical – apply 3-4 times per day and/or after washing.

Nausea

Home remedy.
Calm an upset stomach by rubbing some coconut oil on the inside of arm (from wrist to elbow).

Neuro-degenerative Disorders

Protection against these disorders based on coconut oil's anti-oxidant quality (if disorders are caused by oxidative stress). Management is assisted by ketone supply to the brain.
See Chapter: Research & Promises, specifically Neurodegenerative Disease & Disorders.

Osteoporosis

Research and theory: Coconut oil being used for prevention (possibly treatment) when caused by oxidative bone stress.
Dietary / Preventative.

Pancreatitis

Medium-chain fatty acids do not require pancreatic activity for absorption. Coconut oil helps prevent complications – namely malnutrition and infection.
Dietary / Medicinal – supportive only.

Peptic Ulcer

Stomach ulcers are most often caused by Helicobacter pylori.[52]
Dietary / Medicinal – alternative medicine.
See: Helicobacter pylori

---

52 "What Is Peptic Ulcer Disease?", http://www.webmd.com/digestive-disorders/digestive-diseases-peptic-ulcer-disease

Pneumonia

When cause is viral or bacterial, lauric acid is thought to speed healing in conjunction with antibiotics.
Dietary / Preventative
Dietary / Medicinal - alternative medicine[53]

Pneumonovirus

See Lipid-Coated Virus.

Poison Ivy, Oak, Sumac, Parsnip

Relieves the itch and prevents infection of open wounds. May act as a barrier to prevent spread of toxic plant oils.
Topical – on clean skin as needed.

Prostate Enlargement

Thought to be caused by androgens (male hormones).
Dietary / Preventative.

Psoriasis

Psoriasis can be caused by excessive skin regrowth or it may be immune-mediated. Lauric acid provides relief of inflammation while moisturizing the affected areas.
Topical – daily or as required.

Psoriatic Arthritis

Community support forums occasionally touch on adding dietary coconut oil to help with symptoms of this painful disease.
Current research is contradictory; showing that all fatty acids may aggravate symptoms.[54]
Dietary / Medicinal – home remedy and alternative medicine, proceed with caution.

---

53 Not a research study but a good source of home remedies for the 6th largest killer in America. "Pneumonia Home Remedies", (2013), http://www.kitchenstewardship.com/2013/03/20/do-you-know-two-crazy-symptoms-of-pneumonia-for-toddlers-home-remedies-to-kick-it-without-a-prescription/

Retinopathy

Retina damage and disease. When caused by high blood glucose levels, coconut oil could slow the disease's progression.
Dietary / Preventative.

Rickets

A childhood disease. Coconut oil helps in prevention of rickets caused by malnutrition – mainly insufficient Vitamin D and calcium. Symptom assessment and cures should be managed by a medical practitioner.
Dietary / Preventative – with proper nutrition.

Ringworm

A fungal infection of the skin.
Topical - 5-10 times per day or as needed until healed.

RSV (Human Respiratory Syncytial Virus)

A respiratory tract infection with possibility of recurrence and complication. In adults it can be indistinguishable with the common cold.
See Lipid-Coated Virus.

Sarcoma

See Lipid-Coated Virus.

Shingles

Anti-viral facet of coconut oil relieves the symptoms but also supports the immune system to lessen the risk of return.
Dietary / Preventative – to support immune system.

---

54 "Free fatty acids: potential proinflammatory mediators in rheumatic diseases" (2013)
http://ard.bmj.com/content/early/2013/11/27/annrheumdis-2013-203755.abstract

COCONUT OIL MIRACLE OR MYTH? | 85

Sore Throat

A tablespoon of coconut oil melted in four ounces of warm water. Gargle for 2 minutes.
Dietary / Medicinal - home remedy.

Staph Infection / Staphylococcus aureus / MRSA

A bacterial infection that can manifest in many ways – from pimples to life-threatening diseases that include but are not limited to meningitis and pneumonia. Staph strains are often antibiotic resistant, therefore the best defense is a healthy immune system and cleanliness.
Staphylococcus aureus is a Lipid-Coated Bacterium.
See Lipid-Coated Bacteria.
Dietary / Preventative – to support immune system.

Strep Throat / Streptococcal Tonsillitis / Streptococcal Pharyngitis

Strep is a contagious bacterial infection that left untreated may clear on its own within a few days. Treated with antibiotics, the life of the infection is shortened by a day.
See Lipid-Coated Bacteria.
Dietary / Preventative, Dietary / Medicinal

Stomach Ulcer

See: Peptic Ulcers.

Swimmer's Ear

Caused by bacterial growth in the outer ear canal. Coconut oil eases pressure and controls bacteria.
Topical – a few drops of slightly warmed coconut oil 2-3 times daily until cleared.

Swine Flu

See Lipid-Coated Virus.

Synctial Virus (Human Respiratory Syncytial Virus)

See RSV.

Thrush

An infection of the mouth caused by the candida albicans fungus (aka yeast).
Medicinal.
See Candida Albicans.

Tuberculosis

A highly infectious bacterial disease. Vaccination available. Incidence of infection has increased in the last 10 years. Untreated, patients have a 50% survival rate. Monolaurin has been proven to kill the bacteria in multiple laboratory tests treatment is undocumented or undeveloped.[55]
Unclear, consult a medical professional.

Thyroid Failure

See Hasimoto's.

Ulcerative Colitis

See Digestive Disorder.

Urinary Tract Infection

See Cystitis.

Vaginal Dryness

Could be caused by multiple factors. Common complaint in women over 35.
Topical – daily, to lubricate and moisturize.

Vesicular stomatitis

See Lipid-Coated Virus.

Visna virus

See Lipid-Coated Virus.

---

55 "Preliminary study on the In-Vitro Susceptibility of Mycobacterium tuberculosis Isolates to Virgin Coconut Oil" (2012)
http://functionalfoodscenter.net/files/55970592.pdf

Vitiligo

When caused by oxidative stress, viral or auto-immune
deficiency.
Dietary / Preventative – to support immune system.

Warts / Genital Warts

Caused by a viral infection. Highly contagious. Anti-viral facet of
coconut oil protects against warts but is not effective for
removal.
Topical - use as a moisturizer to protect and prevent spread.

Wounds (skin)

Prevent infection and promote healing.
Topical – immediately, hourly and as needed.

Vaginal Yeast Infection

See Candida Albicans Infection.

Body Weight lbs / kg	Dosage tbsp / day
175+ / 79+	4
150+ / 68+	3 1/2
125+ / 57+	3
100+ / 45+	2 1/2
75+ / 34+	2
50+ / 23+	1 1/2
25+ / 11+	1

How Much To Take?

Disclaimer: These recommendations are not intended to treat, cure or prevent any disease, illness or symptom. Some illnesses and diseases listed above are life threatening. Please consult with your medical practitioner before trying a home remedy. These recommendations are not applicable for pregnant or lactating mothers, or for children.

Antacid – A teaspoon of coconut oil mixed with 1/8 teaspoon of pure cinnamon.

Chemical Detox – Coconut oil's monolaurin attacks toxins in your body. Keep consumption relatively high during an all-body detox.

Insomnia – Better overall health through a balanced diet regulates all body functions, resulting in a better night's sleep.

Healthful Daily Dose

Moments after consumption coconut oil begins ridding your system of toxins, (some) viruses and bacteria, and (some) parasites. Spread consumption into small portions throughout the day.

Start slow and ease into a standard daily dose over the course of 7-10 days. Taking too much, too fast, may cause flu like systems, nausea, rashes or acne. These are standard side effects of any detoxification program.

If you are using coconut oil in your cooking and you are trying to lose weight, cut back on other dietary fats to compensate.

[9]

RESEARCH & PROMISES

Can I get a little personal with you?

As an author, this chapter has been the most difficult to write. I'd like an opportunity to explain why before you being reading. To do so, I have to tell you a little secret about the first book I was commissioned to write.

I had never intended to write a book on any topic. I was a blogger that was scouted and swooned by a large publishing label. That publisher provided the specifications with the contract. When it arrived, so did the advance royalty check that I simply couldn't ignore.

I got right to work and submitted all 60,000 words and photos two days before my deadline.

A week later the manuscript was returned for a rewrite.

I was deflated, then miffed.

My editor requested the hard truths be removed. "Enough of the reality. Sell the dream. Sell the dream and we'll sell the books. Readers will learn the reality and hardships on their own."

Had that been a book on health – quality of life, or life-threatening topics – I would have sent back the advance on royalties and walked away.

This time around I've been very careful with the publishing house I choose.

I can't afford to "sell the dream" when your health might be at stake.

This little book on a simple oil must state the truth, even if the truth is unpopular. I can not chuck ethics and truth aside just to sell a few extra copies of a book.

Tell me what happens when you search the web for coconut oil cures.

Do you see pages of results in Google that read:

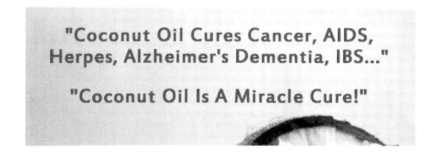

What are all those websites doing? Are they telling you the truth or are they selling the dream?

Sell the dream and sell the books.

Sell the dream and get the clicks.

Selling the dream feeds the family. It keeps the kids in designer labels. It pays the bills.

But it doesn't serve the sick, worried, or the scared.

Spot The Snake Oil

There is one more bit of information I need to share that will help you suss out those who "blow smoke" to make a sale.

On the next page you're going to see the underlying nutrition of a coconut. Not the oil, but the full meat in its raw and natural state.

When you turn the page, don't be dismayed. You already know that our bodies are brilliant in how we put the oil of that meat to use, that it is a speedy and efficient carrier for many nutrients, as well as all the other wonderful anti-microbial virtues.

However, when a coconut is stated as being highly nutritious and rich in fiber, vitamins, and minerals (and this line is pitched all over the internet and in books), consider it a red flag that the entire truth may not follow.

I am not attempting to disrespect authors, journalists, or bloggers but I do have a responsibility to help you uncover the truth.

On the next page you'll see the nutrition data for 1 cup of shredded raw coconut.[56]

I admit it isn't devoid of nutrients, but I'm not certain it could be considered "highly nutritious...rich in vitamins".

---

56 Source: http://caloriecount.about.com/calories-coconut-meat-i12104

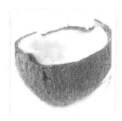

Coconut Meat

Fresh Fruit

coconut, fruit, coconut meat, snack, name this favorite...

B-   283

Grade   Calories

Nutrition Facts

Serving Size 1 cup, shredded (80 g)

Per Serving	% Daily Value*
Calories 283	
Calories from Fat 240	
Total Fat 26.667g	41%
Saturated Fat 23.644g	119%
Polyunsaturated Fat 0.356g	
Monounsaturated Fat 1.067g	
Cholesterol 0mg	0%
Sodium 16mg	0%
Potassium 284mg	9%
Carbohydrates 12.089g	4%
Dietary Fiber 7.111g	28%
Sugars 4.978g	
Protein 2.667g	

Vitamin A 0% · Vitamin C 9%

Calcium 0% · Iron 62%

And although we shouldn't be comparing apples to oranges (in this case coconuts to avocados and almonds) I'm doing so to illustrate a point.

Below and following you'll find the same analysis for 1 cup of mashed avocado,[57] and for 1 cup of raw pistachios.[58]

No matter how you compare a coconut – to a fruit or a nut – it is by no means rich in vitamins.

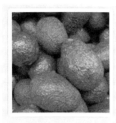

Avocados

Raw, California
avocado, vegetables, fruit, salad, avacado

B+   **384**
Grade   Calories

Nutrition Facts

Serving Size 1 cup, pureed (230 g)

Per Serving	% Daily Value*
Calories 384	
Calories from Fat 319	
Total Fat 35.497g	55%
Saturated Fat 4.919g	24%
Polyunsaturated Fat 4.121g	
Monounsaturated Fat 22.601g	
Cholesterol 0mg	0%
Sodium 19mg	1%
Potassium 1166mg	33%
Carbohydrates 19.809g	7%
Dietary Fiber 15.688g	62%
Sugars 0.665g	
Protein 4.52g	

Vitamin A 7% · Vitamin C 33%
Calcium 3% · Iron 8%

---

57 Source: http://caloriecount.about.com/calories-avocados-i9038

58 Source: http://caloriecount.about.com/calories-pistachio-nuts-i12151

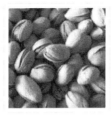

Pistachio Nuts

pistachio nuts, nuts, snack, pistachios, snacks

B	713
Grade	Calories

Nutrition Facts

Serving Size 1 cup (128 g)

Per Serving	% Daily Value*
Calories 713	
Calories from Fat 512	
Total Fat 56.9g	88%
Saturated Fat 7.0g	35%
Polyunsaturated Fat 17.2g	
Monounsaturated Fat 29.8g	
Cholesterol 0mg	0%
Sodium 1mg	0%
Potassium 1312mg	37%
Carbohydrates 35.8g	12%
Dietary Fiber 13.2g	53%
Sugars 9.8g	
Protein 26.4g	

Vitamin A 14% · Vitamin C 11%

Calcium 14% · Iron 30%

[10]

IS COCONUT OIL A MIRACLE CURE?

It is.

And it isn't.

A cure – should it happen – isn't likely to be miracle based solely on coconut oil. It could, however, be a little coconut oil mixed in with plenty of research, hard work and perseverance.

I accept that this truth won't make me popular. I would rather be unpopular than to have a reader become embittered that coconut oil didn't save their son (mother, grandfather, friend). Or distrustful of the medical industry. Or feel that God has turned His back on them.

So here is the truth as I know it. It is based on personal experience, considerable loss, and months of mind-numbing research.

The Truth – As I Know It

I believe in coconut oil. I believe it has restorative powers. I believe it has protective properties and is a powerful antioxidant. More so, I believe everything I have written in this book and already shared with you.

A nutritionist told me something years ago though that I would like to share with you.

"You can consume all the antioxidants, vitamins, good food and miracle cures all day long and it won't make a difference if the rest of your house isn't in order."

The "house" she was talking about was whole health. A house of balanced diet, exercise, gut health, proper hydration and stress management.

The whole health story is seldom told in the miracle claims, testimonials or print books. That is a major disservice to the people who are suffering.

Autoimmune Disorders & Disease

Claims that coconut oil cures autoimmune disorders usually focus on the most common which include but are not limited to Lupus and HIV.

Cure has never been the correct word for any disorder of the immune system. Prevention, perhaps. Supportive after diagnosis, for some.

A similar truth to Steve and Mary's story (see: Neurological & Degenerative Diseases) can apply to every claim of cure or remission once you start digging. Sometimes it shows up more readily – in honest blog posts and books from people who are legitimately trying to share their journey with the world. Other times you have to dig for days just to get past the snake oil.

Many great and humanized (not medical) books have been written on the topic of managing Lupus – but each journey must begin with medical diagnosis and a specialist's care.

HIV+ and HIV-1 are the same. Research suggests that those viruses are compromised in the presence of monolaurin. With regular use, the disease may be manageable through keeping the viral load down. See Chapter: How Monolaurin Kills Lipid-Coated Viruses & Bacteria.

Few people are more excited about this discovery as I am. I have personally watched friends die in the early days of AIDS. More recently I have spent weeks with an associate who worked her life around an HIV infection of over 18 years. Her skin and body look amazing at 42 years of age. She uses coconut oil but she also takes her medications. She has the purest, simplest, and healthiest diet of anyone I know. She exercises daily and she has little outside stress to contend with as her parents and the government pay her bills.

The point is, she doesn't live a normal life and take coconut oil to manage viral load. Her entire life – from sun up to sun down – has zero distractions from pristine health practices.

How many of us can follow such a regime or afford such luxury?

Numerous healing testimonials also abound from doctors and clinics in Malaysia and the Philippines. Two paragraphs at a time we read of cure after cure – but do we ever know the full story?

I accept that coconut oil assists in remission, decreases viral load, and returns people to better health. But like my friend surviving nearly two decades after being diagnosed, there is always more to the story.

Diet, sleep, exercise, stress management – these are the unsung and untold chapters of miracle cures. That, and proof of tenure.

Cancer

Anti-carcinogenic. That is what the literature on coconut oil claims.

I'm about to make a broad sweep, but stick with me, we'll get to some specifics in a few paragraphs.

Worldwide, in all deaths of the year 2007, 13% were caused by cancer – 7.9 million people.[59]

In 2010 in America alone we lost more than 1,500 people a day to cancer.[60]

With all our science and brilliance we're not exactly making progress in combating this disease.

What causes cancer?

Wikipedia states that:
- 30-35% is attributable to diet and obesity
- 25-30% is attributable to smoking
- 15-20% is attributable to infections
- up to 10% is attributable to radiation; and
- 5-10% is attributable to genetics
- ...when added to stress, lack of physical activity and environmental pollutants.

Coconut oil has been proven in a number of in vivo studies to protect the body from breast and colon cancer but more research is required. Prevention is much different than curing, after all.

---

59 "Cancer" Source: http://en.wikipedia.org/wiki/Cancer

60 "Cancer Facts & Figures 2010" American Cancer Society, http://www.cancer.org/research/cancerfactsstatistics/cancerfactsfigures2010/index

A Ground Breaking Book

In 2012, Thomas Seyfried, (a biochemical geneticist who has been investigating the lipid biochemistry of cancer for thirty years), published "Cancer as a Metabolic Disease".

This is a medical textbook written for cancer researchers, clinicians, and public health professionals. It is priced and written above many people's budgets and comprehension – especially those racing to find a cure for a recent prognosis.

I believe the book will be a catalyst for cures in 10-15 years. The review paper, supporting research, and references are available for free online.[61]

To my understanding, the book suggests that cancer can be managed and prevented if it is recognized as a metabolic disease. It also suggests that we can 'starve' those cancer cells through proper diet and weight management. We can also prevent it through the same principles.

Reduce Your Risk by 30-35%

The metabolic disease theory (above) is tightly woven in Western man's glucose consumption. The consumption which has turned to dependence or more correctly described, an addiction.

What if we could break the glucose dependence through a high-fat, moderate-protein, low-carbohydrate diet? What if this diet forced your body to burn stored fat for energy? If we could combat a sugar addiction and remedy obesity, wouldn't it stand to reason that we could decrease our risk of cancer by 30-35%?

That diet – that burns stored fat – is the ketogenic diet. It is also a diet that employs coconut oil as the primary fat source.

---

61 "Cancer As A Metabolic Disease", Thomas N Seyfried and Laura M Shelton, http://www.nutritionandmetabolism.com/content/7/1/7

Remember that the MCFAs in coconut oil is quickly metabolized by the liver into ketones.

Stored fat is burned, the brain and body is still fed, and the problems associated with over-consumption of glucose is solved. It all fits together nicely. The work must still be done, but doing so could add years to your life.

Reduce Your Risk by 15-20%

You have already learned that coconut oil is an anti-microbial that that can remove or protect you from a number of infection causing organisms. As you saw above, an estimated 15-20% of cancers are caused by infections. The culprit is usually a virus, but bacteria and parasites are also causative. Epstein-Barr, HPV, Hep B & C, Helicobacter pylori, Human T-Cell Leukemia – are but a few known to cause cancer.

Diabetes (Type 1 and 2)

It wasn't until Bruce Fife (author and nutritionist) explained the powers of coconut oil for diabetics that I finally understood the disease. Knowing what you have learned so far about the digestion of coconut oil helps to put all the pieces together.

In a non-diabetic person, glucose and fatty acids feed our cells. Without either, cells die and we get sick. When non-diabetics eat, the pancreas creates insulin which carries glucose and fatty acids to the cells.

In Type-1 Diabetes, insulin is not made by the pancreas.

In Type-2 Diabetes, insulin is made by the pancreas, but cells reject it.

Both Type-1 and Type-2 diabetics are prescribed a low-fat diet to keep their need for synthetic insulin minimalized. However, self-managed low-fat diets are often too high in carbohydrates (which require an increase in synthetic insulin) because most of us don't eat enough vegetables. When we're focused on "low-fat", we turn to carbohydrates to satisfy hunger.

Coconut oil is a life-saver for diabetics who have to choose between diet extremes: a strict diet for longevity, or the more satisfying carbohydrate-laden diet with serious health implications.

This is where it gets exciting.

If we can safely add fat to a diabetic's diet, we can make it more satisfying.

If we can safely add fat to a diabetic's diet and it is more satisfying, there is less need to add carbohydrates.

This becomes possible with coconut oil. Where long-chain fatty acids require insulin to be utilized, medium and short chain fatty acids do not. Plus, when those MCFAs enter cells, insulin levels stabilize and little effect is noted on blood glucose levels.

The diabetic's diet becomes far more interesting and satisfying – and vegetables far easier to consume – when a little extra dietary fat is allowed without the need to increase synthetic insulin.

Irritable Bowel Disease & Inflammatory Syndrome

Claims that coconut oil cures these syndromes and diseases focus on Crohn's, ulcerative colitis, diverticulosis, and IBS.

Out of all personal posts in the online communities this is the category where truth, help and honesty are much easier to find. Some would argue that these people aren't fighting for their lives but in a very real sense, they are. People with these intestinal troubles would be on the verge of malnutrition if they didn't manage their intake. Others suffer incredible and consistent pain; all day, every day.

Adding coconut oil to the diet may reduce the painful inflammation, but it doesn't help all sufferers. Again, we're not looking at a cure, we are hoping for help with symptoms and some relief from the complications.

In theory, coconut oil helps through anti-microbial properties. The start of these intestinal troubles is often parasites, bacteria, unresolved viruses, or an overgrowth of yeast.

Not all sufferers know the cause of their disease. Stomach ulcers are often caused by Helicobacter pylori (or another, yet to be defined bacteria) which might affect other areas of the digestive tract. Viruses are being investigated for Crohn's and colitis patients. Some professionals have even theorized that diverticulosis is genetic.

As with any of the serious diseases we have looked at, diet plays a starring role. You will need to be your own hero, learning everything you can along the way. There is ample information to draw from – books and online forums – and new friends to be made that will share their success and their sorrows. To reduce your chance of suffering or further complications, have a medical practitioner providing advice and information.

Neurological & Degenerative Diseases and Disorders

Claims that coconut oil cures neurological and degenerative disorders focus on ALS, Alzheimer's, Autism, Chronic Fatigue, Dementia, and Epilepsy.

In most neurological disorders the brain's ability to use glucose as an energy source has diminished. In these situations, ketones are believed to feed the brain. Coconut oil's fatty acids produce ketones upon digestion.

This method of feeding the brain has been in practice since the early 1920s as the ketogenic diet. It was prescribed to reduce occurrence of seizures in children with epilepsy. The diet helped but didn't meet all dietary needs of growing children. Today the ketogenic diet is followed for adult weight loss and as an at home remedy for neurodegenerative disorders.

To return to the earlier conversation of cures and full disclosure, let's look at a recent news story you might already be familiar with.

Steve Newport and his wife Dr. Mary Newport have been featured on evening news channels and referenced on hundreds of blog articles. Their story is just one of many.

In 2008, at 51 years of age, Steve was diagnosed with Alzheimer's and given medical prescriptions to slow the onset of the disease. All to no avail, none worked and he worsened quickly.

Dr. Mary started him on a coconut oil regime and improvements ensued. His gait returned, his speech improved, and his memory was coming back.

Considering the alternative, which one of us wouldn't gladly take an extra 5 years with an aware spouse? Surely that's worth a few tablespoons of oil every day. Up until the most recent report, this story gave us hope. Steve's remarkable progress received a lot of media attention. It also sold a lot of coconut oil. Five years later, Steve suffered a setback. The prognosis is not hopeful.

The point to ponder is that the full story of his miraculous recovery was not well covered. The full story, according to Dr. Dale Peterson is:

"Steve eats a whole food diet, free of processed foods. He takes 3 tablespoons of a 50/50 mixture of coconut oil and medium chain triglyceride oil three times daily...also takes a teaspoon of cod liver oil and two teaspoons of fish oil daily. His supplements include B vitamins, vitamin C, vitamin E, vitamin D3, niacinamide, turmeric, magnesium, acetyl L-carnitine, coenzyme Q10, D-ribose, phosphatidyl serine, chromium, zinc, and L-lysine. He is also taking two Alzheimer's drugs, Exelon and Namenda."[62]

This looks a lot different than the dream mainstream media is selling us. Imagine the effort and lifestyle changes Steve Newport has undergone in exchange for 5 years of coherency. All worth it, but certainly not a miracle cure.

As I said above: "the miracle could be a little coconut oil mixed in with plenty of research, hard work and perseverance."

---

62 Source:
http://www.drdalepeterson.com/coconut_6297b532e331.shell&print=1

[11]

KITCHEN RECIPES

Blueberry Almond Muffins

These muffins are not the high rising, super sweet, cake-like muffin you'd pick up the local drive through with your morning coffee. They are a nutritious and delicious breakfast muffin that also makes a perfect afternoon snack. Freeze well for up to 4 weeks. If you're on a gluten-free or low carb high fat diet, you'll love these.

Servings: 12
Preparation Time: 15 minutes

1/2 cup	coconut flour
1/2 tsp	baking soda
1/2 tsp	salt
1 cup	bananas, mashed (about 2 medium)
6	eggs, beaten
1 tsp	vanilla extract
	juice from one lemon, zest from ½ lemon
4 tbsp	coconut oil
1/4 cup	sliced almonds, coarsely chopped
1 cup	blueberries

1. Preheat oven to 400ºF.

2. In a large bowl, combine and mix dry ingredients.

3. In a separate bowl, mix bananas with eggs then mix in vanilla, lemon, zest, and coconut oil.

4. Combine banana mixture to dry mixture. Fold in almonds and blueberries.

5. Pour into 12 lightly greased muffin tins and bake for 18 to 20 minutes.

Coconut Oil Granola

4 cups	old-fashioned rolled oats
1 cup	shredded, unsweetened coconut
3/4 cup	raw sunflower seeds
1 1/2 cup	dried fruit (your favorite or a mixture)
1 cup	raw nuts (cashews, pecans or walnuts)
1 tbsp	cinnamon
2 tsp	sea salt
1 tbsp	vanilla extract
1/4 cup	pure maple syrup
1/4 cup	honey
1/4 cup	coconut oil

1. Preheat oven to 250°F.

2. Combine oats, coconut, sunflower seeds, dried fruit, nuts And cinnamon in a large mixing bowl.

3. Over low heat, in a small saucepan, stir together salt, vanilla, maple syrup, honey, and coconut oil until combined.

4. Slowly pour the warm mixture over the dry ingredients while mixing thoroughly to combine.

5. Transfer mixture to a cookie sheet and bake for 40-45 minutes, turning every 15 minutes.

6. Allow to cool completely before transferring to an air tight container.

Notes: I refrigerate my granola out of habit. When purchasing raw nuts and seeds you should always store them in the refrigerator.

Coconut Oil Pound Cake

This loaf style pound cake tastes better than the traditional loaf, even without the butter. Can be eaten warm, but this cake is most flavorful when slightly cooler than room temperatures.

1 cup, plus 2 tbsp	sugar
1/2 cup	virgin coconut oil
3/4 cup	milk
3 large	eggs
1 tsp	vanilla extract
1 3/4 cups	all-purpose flour
2 tsp	baking powder
1/4 tsp	nutmeg
1/4 tsp	salt
1/2 cup	sliced almonds

1. Preheat oven to 350°F.

2. In a saucepan over low heat, warm the coconut oil just to a liquid state. Transfer to a medium mixing bowl and whisk in – one at a time - sugar, milk, eggs and vanilla.

3. In a smaller bowl, whisk together flour, baking powder, nutmeg and salt.

4. Add dry ingredients to the wet ingredients and gently combine. Transfer to a non-stick loaf pan and garnish with almonds.

5. Bake for 45-50 minutes or until the top is golden brown and a toothpick inserted in the center comes out clean. Cool on a wire rack before removing from the pan.

Coconut Oil Vinaigrette

1/4 cup	coconut vinegar
1 tsp	raw honey
1/4 tsp	salt
1/8 tsp	freshly ground black pepper
1/2 cup	coconut oil, liquefied
1/2 cup	virgin olive oil

1. Whisk vinegar, honey, salt and pepper until salt dissolves.
2. Slowly add oils and continue whisking.
3. Allow to stand 5 minutes and serve over crisp salad.

Cornmeal Muffins

A gluten-free, dairy-free, and egg-free version of an American staple. Bake this recipe as a loaf or a muffin, and feel free to add your own nutritious enhancements. If these don't disappear fast enough, they freeze well for up to 4 weeks.

1 cup	cornmeal
1 cup	rice flour
1/2 tsp	salt
4 tsp	baking powder
1 tsp	xanthan gum
1 tbsp	ground flax
1/3 cup	water
1/4 cup	coconut oil at room temperature
1 cup	almond or coconut milk
1/4 cup	honey

1. Preheat oven to 425°F.
2. In a medium bowl, sift together all dry ingredients.
3. In a separate bowl, mix all liquid ingredients

4. Add liquid to the cornmeal mixture and gently stir until just combined.

5. Pour into a lightly greased 8″ square baking dish or greased muffin tins.

6. Bake for 20-25 minutes. Serve warm.

Variations: Adding ½ cup fresh corn and ¼ cup of diced chili makes a nice cornbread for savory meals. Adding ½ cup diced apple and a ¼ cup of dried cranberries make a delicious breakfast when you're running late.

Healthier Mayonnaise

Servings: 1 1/2 cups
Preparation Time: 5 minutes

1	egg
2	egg yolks
1 tbsp	mustard
1 tbsp	fresh lemon juice
1/2 tsp	salt
1/4 tsp	pepper
1/2 cup	coconut oil (melted)
1/2 cup	olive oil

1. Place the eggs, mustard, lemon juice, salt, and pepper into a food processor or blender. Blend briefly for a few seconds.

2. With the processor or blender running on low speed, start adding your oils very slowly. Start out with drops and then work up to about a 1/16″ stream. This will take a few minutes.

3. Continue blending until all the oil is used up and there is no free standing oil.

Healthy Sweet Potato Fries

Servings: 6
Preparation Time: 10 minutes

4-5	medium sweet potatoes, wedged
3 tbsp	warmed coconut oil
1/2 tsp	salt
2 tsp	chopped fresh garlic
1/2 tsp	freshly grated black pepper
	any other favorite spice or herb

1. Preheat oven to 425°F.

2. In a large bowl combine all ingredients and stir until sweet potato wedges are uniformly coated.

3. Arrange in a single layer on cookie sheets and bake for 30-45 minutes until cooked and slightly crispy (30-40 minutes dependent on size of wedge).

Dirty Spiced Rice

Servings: 8
Preparation Time: 25-30 minutes

2 tbsp	coconut oil
4 cloves	garlic, crushed
½ tsp	chili pepper flakes
1 tbsp	fresh ginger, grated
2 cups	brown rice
3/4 cup	coconut milk
3 cups	water

1. In a medium saucepan, lightly sauté garlic and ginger in coconut oil.

2. Add rice and stir for 1 minute, then add remaining ingredients.

3. Quickly bring the rice to a boil, stirring often, and reduce heat.

4. Cover, simmer, and stir occasionally for 25-30 minutes or until done.

5. Remove from heat and allow the rice to rest for 5 minutes or more before serving.

Zucchini Bread

3	eggs, beaten
2 cups	white sugar
1 cup	coconut oil (warmed)
2 cups	raw zucchini, unpeeled and grated
2 cups	all purpose flour
¼ tsp	baking powder
2 tsp	baking soda
1 tsp	salt
2 tsp	cinnamon
2 tsp	vanilla
3/4 cup	chopped pecans (or any nut - optional)

1. Preheat oven to 350°F.

2. In a medium mixing bowl, beat eggs, sugar and coconut oil 1-2 minutes until creamy. Stir in zucchini.

3. In a separate bowl, mix flour, baking soda, baking powder, salt, and cinnamon.

4. Fold the flour blend into the first bowl, mixing well.

5. Pour into two non-stick small loaf pans and bake 40-45 minutes.

6. Serve warm or cold. Freezes well for up to a month.

[12]

PERSONAL CARE RECIPES

Body Scrub / Skin Exfoliation

A spa-like micro-dermabrasion treatment for your arms, legs and back.

Mix equal parts of coconut oil and sugar – you may need to warm up the coconut oil slightly to mix it together.

1. Experiment with all types of sugar until you find the one you like the best; brown sugar will be the quickest to dissolve and works best for sensitive skin types.

2. Jazz up your scrub with a few drops of your favorite essential oil. After you rinse off, your skin will be soft, refreshed and protected. Extra sugar can be added for a denser scrub.

Cuticle Cream / Cuticle Remover

Rub small amounts of coconut oil into dry cuticles to moisturize plus to prevent or treat hangnails. Before a manicure, rub slightly warmed coconut oil into the base of each nail to soften cuticles for removal.

Eyelash / Brow Conditioner

When moisturizing your face, don't forget to lightly moisturize brows and lashes. Coconut oil strengthens and thickens both.

Facial Cleanser

Traditional soap is little more than lye, fats and a few fragrances. Take advantage of coconut oil's natural anti-bacterial and anti-fungal properties and use it straight from the jar to wash your face. It will remove make-up, oils and environmental impurities.

If you feel you need a little more abrasion, make your own facial scrub by mixing a little brown sugar with warmed coconut oil in a small jar. To use either, gently massage coconut oil or scrub into face for 1-2 minutes, then rinse off with warm water.

Hair Dye Repellant

Stylists use a petroleum-based oil to protect face, neck and ears from hair dye. Coconut oil works equally well.

Hand Sanitizer

Hand sanitizers are drying and (according to recent studies) are not good for the environment. You can easily make your own from 2 easy-to-find, all natural ingredients that kill germs and bacteria.

Mix 10 drops of oil of oregano to four tablespoons of slightly warmed coconut oil and transfer to a jar with a tight-fitting lid. Keep it in your purse or pocket but remember that at 76 degrees that oil will melt. Apply repeatedly throughout the day, especially after you have been in public places.

Home Made Body Deodorant

Commercial deodorants have a lot of bad press for good reasons. Coconut oil, applied directly to underarms, prevents bacteria and fungi, the two main causes of body odor.

Aluminum-free, all natural with the added benefit of coconut oil's antibacterial and anti-fungal properties. Perfect for sensitive skin.

- 2 tbsp coconut oil
- ½ cup baking soda
- ½ cup cornstarch or arrowroot powder
- ½ tsp essential oil (citrus, mint, lavender – your favorite)

Warm coconut oil until it is a liquid state and mix in remaining ingredients.

The deodorant will firm back up once it cools down so you'll want to store it in a wide mouthed jar.

Only a small amount is required per use (apply as much as you would if it was a moisturizer). Apply as often as needed.

Makes about 12 ounces – enough for 4-8 weeks depending on usage.

Note: If you are converting to a holistic diet you may find that once blockages and toxins have been removed from your body, perspiration neither stinks nor stains clothing and you can go without deodorant of any sort. Continue to moisturize your underarms with coconut oil.

Home Made Toothpaste

A mix of coconut oil and baking soda provides enough abrasion plus anti-bacterial agents to clean and strengthen teeth and gums, plus keep bad breath at bay.

One small (2-3 ounce) jar will last 3-4 weeks. Use about 1/10 the amount of a commercially prepared toothpaste per brushing.

- Equal parts coconut oil and baking soda.

1. Warm coconut oil until liquid state and mix in an equal amount of baking soda.
2. Place in a wide-mouthed jar so you can easily scoop it out as required.

Insect Repellent

Make a non-toxic repellent by mixing 10-12 drops of an essential oil into ½ cup of coconut oil and store in a jar by the door. Rub it into all exposed skin before going outside. It moisturizes your skin and repels pesky bugs.

Essential oils, in order of effectiveness against bugs are: citronella[63], clove, rosemary, geranium, lemongrass, tea tree, eucalyptus, cedar, thyme.

Lip Balm

Don't forget your lips when moisturizing your face, neck and decollette with coconut oil. I keep a small jar of coconut oil in my

---

63 Direct application of citronella oil has been found to raise the heart rate of some people.[10] Health Canada is in the process of phasing out citronella entirely, as an insect repellent.[11] The EPA, on the other hand, finds no known toxicity for citronella. Source: http://en.wikipedia.org/wiki/Citronella_oil

purse so I can reapply throughout the day but only when average temperatures are below 70 degrees F as I've had more than one instance of oil turning to its liquid state and leaking over my checkbook.

Moisturizer – All Skin Types

Your skin always requires moisture to remain healthy, even if it is naturally oily. After a few weeks of use you might even find that your skin balances itself out and stops excessive oil production.

Sexual Lubricant

Coconut oil, in its natural state, it is an all-natural sexual lubricant. Not compatible with latex condoms.

Shaving Cream & Aftershave

Coconut oil can replace shaving cream as well as aftershave. As an aftershave it moisturizes face, leg and underarm skin while protecting freshly shaved skin from bacteria.

Sunscreen

As is, coconut oil is a very light sunscreen, offering an SPF between 4-6.

Quick List

Twenty five coconuts yield one quart of virgin coconut oil.

The average adult coconut palm will grow 45 coconuts/year.

Coconut oil:

- Has an approximate shelf life of 2 years.

- Does not need to be refrigerated.

- Should be kept out of direct sunlight.

- Solid turns to oil at 76 °F, 24 °C.

- Warms/melts quickly in your palm.

- Has 0 (zero) glycemic load. The glycemic index is a method of measuring the impact of foods on blood sugar.

- Has 130 calories per tablespoon.

Smoke Points:

- virgin coconut oil, 350°F/177°C

- refined coconut oil, 450°F/232°C

Recommended Reading

ALS

- Surviving Without Your MD: Do Prescription Drugs Ever Cure? by Eric Edney and Glenna Edney

- Eric Is Winning: Beating a Terminal Illness with Nutrition, Avoiding Toxins and Common Sense by Eric Edney

Ayurvedic Medicine

- The Complete Book of Ayurvedic Home Remedies by Vasant Masc Lad

Coconut Oil

- Coconut Oil Nutrition Book by Patrick Smith

- The Coconut Oil Miracle by Bruce Fife

Fats & Oils

- Fats That Heal, Fats That Kill by Udo Erasmus

Printed in Great Britain
by Amazon.co.uk, Ltd.,
Marston Gate.